Giorgio Repeti,
with Marc S. Micozzi, MC,

Wan's CLINICAL
APPLICATION OF
CHINESE MEDICINE

Scientific Practice of Diagnosis,
Treatment and Therapeutic Monitoring

SINGING
DRAGON

LONDON AND PHILADELPHIA

First published in 2011
by Singing Dragon
an imprint of Jessica Kingsley Publishers
116 Pentonville Road
London N1 9JB, UK
and
400 Market Street, Suite 400
Philadelphia, PA 19106, USA

www.singing-dragon.com

Library of Congress Cataloging in Publication Data
A CIP catalog record for this book is available from the Library of Congress

British Library Cataloguing in Publication Data
A CIP catalogue record for this book is available from the British Library

ISBN 978 1 84819 047 4

Printed and bound in the United States
by Thomson-Shore, Inc.

Wan's CLINICAL APPLICATION OF CHINESE MEDICINE

of related interest

Chinese Medical Qigong
Editor in Chief: Tianjun Liu, O.M.D.
Associate Editor in Chief: Kevin W Chen, Ph.D.
Foreword by Marc Micozzi, M.D., Ph.D.
ISBN 978 1 84819 023 8

Basic Theories of Traditional Chinese Medicine
Edited by Zhu Bing and Wang Hongcai
Advisor: Cheng Xinnong
ISBN 978 1 84819 038 2

Diagnostics of Traditional Chinese Medicine
Edited by Zhu Bing and Wang Hongcai
Advisor: Cheng Xinnong
ISBN 978 1 84819 036 8

Meridians and Acupoints
Edited by Zhu Bing and Wang Hongcai
Advisor: Cheng Xinnong
ISBN 978 1 84819 037 5

Acupuncture Therapeutics
Edited by Zhu Bing and Wang Hongcai
Advisor: Cheng Xinnong
ISBN 978 1 84819 039 9

Case Studies from the Medical Records of Leading Chinese Acupuncture Experts
Edited by Zhu Bing and Wang Hongcai
Advisor: Cheng Xinnong
ISBN 978 1 84819 046 7

Celestial Healing
Energy, Mind and Spirit in Traditional Medicines of China and East and Southeast Asia – Greater China
Marc S. Micozzi
ISBN 978 1 84819 060 3

To Grandmaster Yuen Tung

Fortunate is the one who receives the Teaching
Fortunate is the one who is One pointed of Mind
Fortunate is the one who understands the Dhamma

Disclaimer

Every effort has been made to ensure that the information contained in this book is correct, but it should not in any way be substituted for medical advice. Readers should always consult a qualified medical practitioner before adopting any complementary or alternative therapies. Neither the author nor the publisher takes any responsibility for any consequences of any decision made as a result of the information contained in this book.

CONTENTS

List of Figures and Tables

ABOUT THE AUTHOR

Giorgio Repeti is a licensed acupuncturist who studied under Dr. Wan, the founder of the 3E Method, from 1992 until his death in 1997. He also studied under Dr. Liew, in the Hannya ShangYi (Wise Superior Method) from 1992 to 2003.

From 1998 to 2003 he attended the University of New South Wales and the University of Western Sydney, Sydney, Australia, to earn a Bachelor of Applied Science (Traditional Chinese Medicine). He worked in a drug and alcohol rehabilitation center in Moree, New South Wales, Australia, for over two years, one of few acupuncturists to be admitted to practice in such a facility. He also founded and directed the Everest College of Natural Medicine in Sydney for six years and was a contributor to the textbook *Purple Healer* by Mark Nicholson, with a chapter entitled "Basic Pulse Palpation."

He came to the U.S. in 2004 and in 2005 passed the board exam under The National Certification Commission for Acupuncture and Oriental Medicine in the United States and became licensed to practice acupuncture in New York. Giorgio also worked at the Eastchester Center for Cancer Care in the Bronx, New York, for a year, being one of very few acupuncturists to have had the opportunity to work in such a clinical setting.

He subsequently maintained a private practice in New York City and for two years served on the board of the Acupuncture Society of New York.

EDITOR'S PREFACE

Much acupuncture practice in the West is incomplete or incorrect because it has been based upon particular interpretations, often accounting for only part of the rich corpus available from the ancient Chinese classics. The result is a somewhat watered down version which is less potent than might otherwise be achieved in many clinical situations. When therapeutic problems are encountered with a particular condition, or in a particular individual, too often there is an inability to pursue the next steps by consulting the real solutions to these clinical problems that are available but have hitherto been hidden in the Chinese medical classics for "difficult issues."

Added to this is the reality that the "secrets" of specific therapeutic techniques are passed down by generations of practitioners, from master to student and disciple. What is presented to the ordinary person is only partial knowledge, and what is given to the student is not the same as what the master will pass on to the true disciple. According to Master Wan, here are the particulars of clinical practice moving from the classic sources to the bedside.

Thus, these techniques can be used to actually monitor the effects of treatments in real time. This is not the same as inserting needles and walking away from the patient to attend to something else. The author provides these secrets of Master Wan, together with the basics of diagnosis and treatment in easily accessible form.

Chinese medicine and acupuncture has more to offer, for more people, with more clinical conditions, than has generally been available in the state of practice in the contemporary West. This book goes a long way to place more powerful tools in the hands of practitioners and to expand our knowledge of the full potential of Chinese medical practices.

Because this book has been designed as a handy clinical manual, those seeking for a deeper background in the scholarship and theories of Chinese medicine may find it works best as a companion book to other basic, comprehensive texts on Chinese medicine and acupuncture. It makes a good "pocket guide" for those wanting a handy reference, a short basic review, and a practical hands-on guide.

Marc S. Micozzi, MD, PhD

INTRODUCTION:
HOW TO USE THIS BOOK

Guru Yuen Tung—Grandmaster Dr. Wan, was phenomenal in his wisdom, knowledge and depth of clinical experience as Founder of the Lingsu practice. He was also known by the title His Holiness, and was well versed in Taoism and Buddhism.

Grandmaster Wan was my main teacher and the source for this book, although it also pays homage to *all* my teachers. Grandmaster Wan shows us the possibility and practicality of quick and clinically effective results from the use of very few points. I did not think this was possible until I observed him in practice. He called his acupuncture and Chinese medicine method 3E (I will explain this later in detail).

In this book, through his student, Grandmaster Wan's wisdom is brought to life. The 3E Method provides clear diagnostic tools, acupuncture practices using few points, and abbreviated herbal formulas for more practical effectiveness. This text will help to keep the 3E Method alive, as Grandmaster Wan did not teach many students. Since Dr. Wan's death in July 1997, I have taken on the challenge to formulate his teaching in a concise, easy to understand format. Much of his diagnostic component remains unchanged.

The acupuncture needling and herbal protocols have been recorded systematically as the teaching was received. (He taught the needling and the prescription method more practically, and not so often in the 'classroom' setting.) Much of Dr. Wan's teaching style is hands-on learning through observation, silence, and finally investigating the teaching and the Method through intense practice. After Dr. Wan died I completed my theoretical training under Dr. Liew who at that time was developing the 3E Method. However, he changed the name from 3E Method to "Hannya ShangYi Physician Course," and called the herbal component "Herbal Holistic," using the term "Naturoherbs." In light of this, when I began to compile the Method in 1998 I confronted the temptation to change the direct teaching of Dr. Wan, to make it my own point of view. After considering my responsibility to future students I realized that I was, in essence, like a radio transmitter allowing the information to pass through on my bandwidth and nothing much else. I also realized that to change the already perfected theoretical knowledge after Dr. Wan's painstaking four decades of practice would indeed be unjust.

Therefore I humbly present the teaching in the original form with minimal interference, although it was necessary to make the flow of information "logical." The Method was taught to me in cafés, at dinner and lunch in restaurants, whilst driving, in the clinic, in the classroom, out on walks, after meditation, and generally in the midst of life. It was necessary to structure the teaching in an easy, logical flowing context.

In Dr. Wan's tradition the adept needs to breathe, eat, sleep, and even dream the Method! Dr. Wan was an intensive teacher, but also made clear the necessity to be relaxed, poised, and calm while studying, investigating, and applying the Method. Self-awareness is key in the practice of Wan's 3E Method.

3E principles

Fundamentals

Wan used few points in treatment—this to me actually represents an important advance in the field of acupuncture. Most texts today talk about using many points (sometimes over 20 at a time), and there are a proliferating number of books about them. Yet Dr. Wan insisted that good understanding in acupuncture therapy requires the use of *few* points in treatment.

I would like to share an experience from many years ago whilst I was at a First Aid course in Sydney at the Red Cross building near Wynyard Station. The teacher shared a story with the class that has remained in my thinking till this day.

That instructor liked to fail "Advanced first aid students," not by providing them with complicated tests or trickery *but* by simply reissuing the "basic" first aid exam! A majority of the students would usually fail! This lesson represents an important point. "In complication, we need to stick with the basics first," is to me a Golden Rule and in my experience has been incomprehensibly important. (And, yes, I failed that exam too!)

Stay with the fundamentals. They will not fail you. And keep it simple. The same is true in science. An early Nobel laureate once said, "If you need statistics to understand the result of your experiment, you should have done a better experiment."

In my practice I have tried many theories and fundamentals and have found simplicity to be the most effective form of therapy. Simplicity requires deep understanding of the fundamentals and the ability to do less to have a more profound effect. This theory operates in many areas of our lives, however, in acupuncture, the understanding that "energy" has purpose and directions needs to be fixed in one's mind. For this "energy," when *not* achieving its purpose, creates a blockage often resulting in pain, injury, disease, and even premature death. This purposeful energy needs to reclaim its direction and intent, which is the aim of acupuncture therapy in Dr. Wan's model. When the energy flow, wherever it may be, is suppressed, blocked, or hindered, symptoms result.

The purpose of fewer needles

Imagine getting directions when you are in a state of panic—are you likely to be able to follow one or two simple instructions, or 10 or 12? Imagine an acupuncture point—one point can have a myriad of functions. If one point has at least five functions or actions, and we stimulate ten points, we are in fact eliciting a possible fifty actions or functions. In fact, physiologically we may envision it as having 50! (50 factorial, that is, $50 \times 49 \times 48 \times 47 \ldots \times 3 \times 2 \times 1$) effects.

For example, someone has pain in a location like the elbow. Depending upon the severity of the pain the patient may be in a state where the emotions, mind, and body are tense, stressed, or weak. In this state would it be wiser to give the mind and body fifty directions or five (let alone 50 factorial)?

Efficiency is "doing less to do more" is it not? In Wan's 3E Method we propose that in a state of illness, shock, pain, weakness, the body itself, being highly complex, responds to simple and straightforward direction. Saturating the body with too many messages can be overwhelming to the brain and body and may even hinder healing.

Alarm stage of pathogenesis

In the alarm state of pathogenesis, clear direct signals are best to quell and harmonize the panic and turn it into whatever effective actions are required. Most treatments revolve around doing more in the panic stage, however, it is my opinion that doing less, but giving a clear direct signal gives rise to more efficiency and overall has a much deeper effect in calming the body.

For example, in shock: what is the most effective treatment? Lie the person down and raise the legs and apply warmth—this is pure mechanics, letting gravity bring blood flow back to the Heart and brain, and conserving heat. Then proceed with whatever treatment is necessary, however the shock needs to be dealt with first, that's the point.

This simple scenario is not always the case, and this book does not in any way simplify treatment of disease, nor the treatment of shock. However it is stressed that the approach needs to be simple and straightforward, with strong and correct fundamentals.

Lastly, nothing in this book has been added just for the sake of appearances. Every word has been thought about extensively, every chapter has been written with serious intent and strategy, to give the reader a flowing, harmonious, and easy way to study and apply the Method.

Wan's 3E Method is unique

To practice legally in Sydney, Australia, and later on in Manhattan, New York it was mandatory to complete a Bachelor of Science (TCM) degree to formalize my studies, as Dr. Wan and Dr. Liew's training was not accredited by the government, and so was not recognized as an official qualification.

Throughout my studies at the University of Western Sydney, Australia, under well-versed teachers it started to become clear that Wan's 3E Method was unique and not well known in the major circles of TCM in Australia. What further highlighted to me the uniqueness of the 3E Method was my visit to Nanjing, China, Hong Kong, and various clinics in New York. I saw no evidence of Wan's 3E Method format, its principles, and treatment strategies. Dr. Wan had handfuls of students in Germany, Japan, and in other parts of the world but there is no record of where or who they all are.

When I was studying for the "official" board exam in New York in 2005 I saw little similarity to Wan's 3E diagnostic method for the tongue and even less for his pulse diagnosis. I saw no relation or similarity in the use of few acupuncture points in treatment, and the herbal and needling methods were not seen in any of the suggested texts, except of course, for the obvious, tonification and sedation methods in the needling method and use of points. It seemed that Wan's 3E Method had been lost to the official regulators of Chinese medicine, or never discovered.

One text with similar theory, but not treatments, is *Golden Needle Wang Le Ting*[1] (Hui Chan Yu and Fu Ru Han 1997). One of the major points that is consistent between Wang Le Ting's theories and Wan's 3E Method is the suggestion that there is no "Neutral" or "Even" method of needling, but there is either "Tonification" or "Sedation." Another text with the same view is *A Study of Daoist Acupuncture and Moxibustion* (Cheng Tsai Liu, Liu Zheng Cai and Ka Hua 1999). It also has similarities in treatment fundamentals such as time for tonification and sedation, and other needling methods.

On the topic of pulse I found that Huang Fu Mi's book (2007, Chapter 1), captures the essence of Dr. Wan's Ren Ying and Cun Kou methods. However, after learning the 3E Method of Ren Ying and Cun Kou from Dr. Wan and later from Dr. Liew, I noticed a fundamental difference in Huang Fu Mi's diagnosis and treatment formulations.

A new system?

Is it possible that Dr. Wan had discovered or rediscovered an old system? Or is it a new system, entirely emanating from his wisdom? I continue to study and attend seminars in New York, and have found no evidence of it being an old system—other than similarities in the texts already mentioned. While Wan's 3E Method does appear to flow from his wisdom it cannot be known for certain whether he once used any of the above texts in their original Chinese versions. However, we know that he definitely could not have used these texts in English as he created the 3E Method in the 1960s, long before any of them were translated and published in English.

---

1   Wang Le Ting was an acupuncture practitioner in the mid twentieth century. He is widely considered to be one of the architects of modern Chinese acupuncture as he created many new treatment protocols that are useful in the treatment of chronic conditions.

So the question remains, but it is not as important as the 3E Method itself. We are only faced with the goal of bringing it to the world.

Original teaching

I have noted in the text where my own input and experience is expressed so that there is no confusion with Wan's authentic 3E Method. I have added a fundamental philosophical discussion to the application of healing in general, and took the liberty to suggest some practices the practitioner should be doing on a personal level as well. When Dr. Wan died there was very little written down about the "whole" practice so this text can be considered the first to be released publicly.

Wan's 3 Es

Now for the mystery of the 3 Es in Wan's 3E Method: Easy, Economical, and Efficient. Dr. Wan insisted that any good therapy must contain these three ingredients. An old aphorism in the West, often repeated to the editor, both as student and colleague, by a former U.S. Surgeon General is "the least medicine that works is the best medicine."

- Efficiency in diagnosis, Efficiency in treatment
- Easy to see, Easy to apply
- Economical in delivery, fewer needles, work, time and herbs

The 3 Es will be expanded upon throughout the text.

The text is a living teaching

The way to get maximum benefit from the text is for the reader to visualize being in a clinical situation when reading, and utillizing the text as if a teacher were guiding their practice. Every teaching in the text is to be applied and then observed, not just thought about. This is crucial. It is a waste of time to ask mechanistic questions such as "why" in the beginning. Through practice and careful application the reader will eventually understand.

The book can be read repeatedly over many years. Eventually the reader will realize the extent of the detail of the teaching and how advanced it really is. This is not a book to be read once or to be taken lightly. It is a living teaching of a unique method.

The way of Tao

It is interesting to note the various styles of acupuncture and Chinese herbal prescriptions that exist in the world of traditional Chinese, Japanese, Korean, and Vietnamese medicine. The variety is often overwhelming. The information is vast, and hard to navigate. For the practitioner it becomes a huge task to search through all the texts. This book was written with the clinician in mind; to set the parameters of observation after learning the foundation theory.

In a seminar conducted by Giovanni Maciocia in New York on May 17–18, 2008, it was interesting to note the differences in Taoist and Confucianist thought and practice. He expressed and discussed the differences between the Confucian texts that speak about the body needing to be *controlled*, in expressions such as "attack the Qi," "control the flow," versus the Taoist fundamental that the body is a perfect entity that can redirect and heal itself. It is often forgotten that there are differences between the Confucianist and the Taoist schools of thought in terms of application of acupuncture therapy. This text intends to clarify this distinction.

- The body is perfect—humans are perfect, nature is perfect. Nothing needs to be controlled—nature balances itself, to think that the Creator did not consider balance in his creations is not correct thinking.

  □ The body is perfect.

  □ Perfect in design.

☐ Perfect in function.

- Acupuncture manipulates and helps direct the body's own natural energy to heal itself.

- Everything on earth has its own flow, coming and going, beginning and end. The human body has a lifespan and its natural direction is to break down, as the natural direction of everything is entropy.

Lineage of practitioners

I feel a duty to reach all those interested in Chinese medicine around the world, with the intention that this rare method will continue to be available via this text and that adepts will keep it in its pure form and resist changing something that works so profoundly. Nothing needs to be updated or changed. It is perfect as it is. It is the responsibility of future students to keep the teaching intact.

The role of teacher

When I started writing this text back in 1998 my experience was short in the application of Wan's 3E Method so I decided to record my observations, epiphanies, and struggles along the way. We present here 12 years of effort with all the collated information and struggles with various problems of accuracy. There is the ever present danger of the reader misunderstanding the teaching.

In the best of all possible worlds it would be advantageous to have access to a well-versed teacher of Wan's 3E Method to help explain the text to you. For most people this is not possible and therefore this text has been written.

We hope it is presented in such a way, that you can investigate the Method, apply it, monitor it, and experience the intended results. Like any good read, you will come back to the text again and again. Use it for a period of 3–5 years for the best results. Be a scientist, investigate and apply.

This text is primarily presented for a reader with a bachelor's degree in Chinese medicine, or a related degree, and at least a few years of clinical experience. The text is clinically based. Dr. Wan's 3E Method is profound and can help lead the practitioner from Mastery to the "Superior" level physician spoken about in the *Yellow Emperor's Inner Classic*, or *Canon of Internal Medicine*.

To the master, teacher, and practitioner

I hope you enjoy and find interesting the following compilation of clinical explanation and theory and that this text inspires you to learn, investigate, and apply Wan's unique 3E Method. May it improve your therapy and your service to your patients.

To the student

It is important for a student to feel, see, and experience results from diagnosis and therapy. As a student it is important to believe in one's teacher (as is the old custom); however, belief is only the first step. Results build credibility and are imperative for growth towards the final steps of mastering the practice. If the results are not felt, seen, and experienced then it is blind faith—not appropriate for the scientist.

In some schools the emphasis is based on trusting the teacher as the main focus. In Wan's 3E Method the student can believe in the teacher at first, but then needs to see, feel, and experience the results as proof of the teaching. This is the scientific method of practice. Do not let theories get in the way of observing practical results.

To the general reader

We have presented the role of belief in the world of the teachers and students. For anyone interested in the great healing traditions of Asia, this book reveals many secrets that have never before been made known.

1

WAN'S 3E DIAGNOSTIC METHOD

Introduction

The following information is included here to give the reader a concise review of the many diagnostic tools used in Chinese medicine, including:

- Yin and Yang principles
- the Five Elements
- examination of the six types of body syndrome
- eye diagnosis
- facial diagnosis
- pulse diagnosis
- tongue diagnosis.

The following are not included:

- abdomen palpation (Hara diagnosis)
- asking
- listening and smelling.

Dr. Wan's summation of the above-mentioned methods of diagnosis follows. It is good practice to briefly refresh our memory from time to time with the fundamentals. Without the correct understanding and absorption of the right fundamentals the practice will be sub-standard. Wan's 3E Method helps maintain the standard, and a correct understanding of the fundamentals is key to engaging better future practice.

Yin and Yang principles

Diagnosis and prescribing are based on Yin and Yang.

A state of health is maintained when there is balance between Yin and Yang.

Excess of one automatically leads to the depletion of the other. It is excess that is noticed, while deficiency can go unnoticed.

There are several basic relationships or conditions of Yin and Yang. The model describing them can help form the basis for diagnosis and treatment.

The thick line in Figure 1.1 is the line of balance, or midpoint, which indicates homeostasis. The (+) or Yang side represents and is manifested by heat, action, Fire, energy, Qi. The (–) side, or Yin, represents and is manifested by cold, inaction, stasis, water, blood.

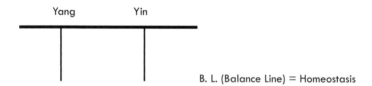

Figure 1.1: The basic condition of balance, where both Yin and Yang are just right

Figure 1.1 represents the basic condition of balance, where both Yin and Yang are just right.

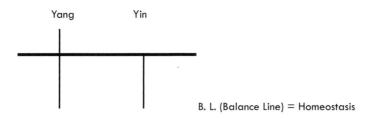

Figure 1.2: A situation where the Yang is excessive

Figure 1.2 represents a situation where the Yang is excessive. This excess can manifest in heat and/or inflammation. The way to deal with this imbalance is to reduce the excess Yang. Western medicine will use antibiotics and aspirin.

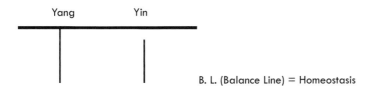

Figure 1.3: A condition of Yin deficiency

The condition represented by Figure 1.3 is of Yin deficiency. In this case we must tonify or replenish the Yin.

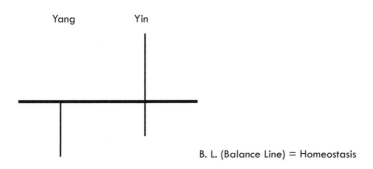

Figure 1.4: A condition of excess Yin

The condition represented by Figure 1.4 is one of excess Yin. This condition is actually very rare. Even here we do not try to diminish the Yin because the saying in Chinese medicine is "Yin is always insufficient." For example, we can just give a bit of ginger to counteract the coldness.

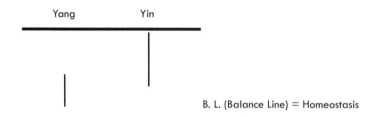

Figure 1.5: A condition of deficient Yang

Figure 1.5 represents a condition of deficient Yang. In this case we must replenish the Yang.

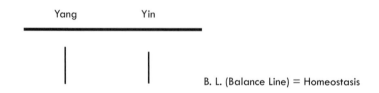

Figure 1.6: A condition of deficient Yang and Yin

Figure 1.6 represents a condition of deficient Yang and Yin. In this case we must replenish both. This condition is one of general debility or weakness.

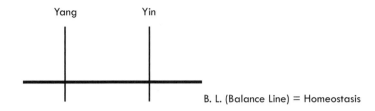

Yang   Yin

B. L. (Balance Line) = Homeostasis

Figure 1.7: A theoretical condition with excess of both Yin and Yang

Figure 1.7 shows a theoretical condition with excess of both Yin and Yang and is seldom encountered.

The Five Elements

Chinese medicine diagnosis can be better understood and memorized using the rudimentary Five Elements Theory. The Five Elements are Fire, Earth, Metal, Water, and Wood.

The Five Elements maintain two basic relationships between them. These relationships manifest in the interactions between them and are important in determining the prognosis of the patient.

The first relationship is that of mother and child. In other words, each element nourishes or produces another element as follows:

- Fire produces Earth.

- Earth produces Metal.

- Metal produces Water.

- Water produces Wood.

- Wood produces Fire.

The second relationship is that of antagonizing or controlling. In other words, each element acts against another element as follows:

- Fire antagonizes (melts) Metal.

- Metal antagonizes (cuts) Wood.

- Wood antagonizes (depletes) Earth.

- Earth antagonizes (soaks) Water.

- Water antagonizes (puts out) Fire.

Both relationships of nourishing and antagonizing can be summarized in Figure 1.8.

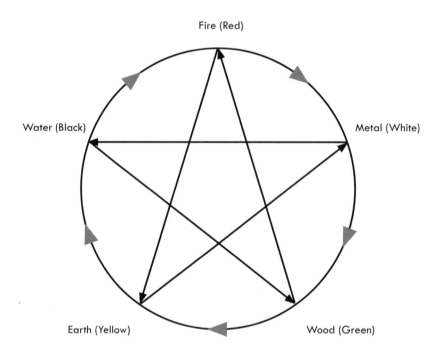

→	Represents: nourishing, creating—tonifying
▲	Represents: antagonising, controlling—sedating

Figure 1.8: The Five Elements; nourishing and antagonizing relationships

Table 1.1 The Five Elements

Nature								Body					
Direction	Taste	Color	Energy	Environmental factor	Season	Element		Zang	Fu		Five sense organs	Five tissues	Emotions
East	Sour	Green	Germination	Wind	Spring	Wood		Liver	Gb		Eyes	Tendon	Anger
South	Bitter	Red	Growth	Heat	Summer	Fire		Heart	Si		Tongue	Blood vessels	Laughter
Center	Sweet	Yellow	Transformation	Dampness	Late summer	Earth		Spleen	St		Mouth and lips	Muscles	Thinking
West	Pungent	White	Gathering	Dryness	Autumn	Metal		Lung	Li		Nose	Skin and hair	Grief, sadness
North	Salty	Black	Storage	Cold	Winter	Water		Kidney	Bl		Ears	Bone	Fear, fright

Table 1.2 Body fluids

Element	Secretion
Wood	Tears
Fire	Sweat
Earth	Saliva
Metal	Mucus
Water	Urine

Table 1.3 Grains and sounds

Element	Sounds	Characteristics	Grain
Wood	Knock on wood	Shouting	Legumes
Fire	Hissing	Laughing	Rye/wheat
Earth	Hit on ceramic	Pensiveness	Rice
Metal	Twang twang	Crying	Millet
Water	Crystal sounds	Yawning	Beans

Combining the various diagnostic techniques

In Chinese medicine the diagnostic process consists of the following elements:

- observation
- listening and smelling
- asking
- abdomen palpation
- facial diagnosis (see p.36)
- pulse diagnosis (see p.40)

- eye diagnosis (see p.45)

- tongue diagnosis (see p.47).

A reliable diagnosis can only be made by combining all of these methods. For any indication that we get using one method we should immediately look for corroborating or contradicting indications using the other methods before making the final diagnosis.

The Five Organs diagnostic technique

Each of the Five Organs is related to one of the Five Elements as follows:

- Fire   =   Heart

- Earth   =   Spleen

- Metal   =   Lungs

- Water   =   Kidneys

- Wood   =   Liver

We will not talk specifically about the five Fu organs individually since they relate to the organs in pairs (e.g. Spleen and Stomach form a pair).

Table 1.4 The Zang-Fu organs

Zang	Fu
Lung	Large Intestine
Kidney	Bladder
Liver	Gallbladder
Heart	Small Intestine
Spleen	Stomach

Qi: Life-force (vital) energy levels

Table 1.5 Life-force domains—the five Qi domains of the body

Heavenly Qi—life-force	Produced in the Lungs
Primordial Qi—life-force	Produced from Jing—essence
Protective Qi—life-force	Moving around the body
Congenital Qi—life-force	Inherited from parents
Nutrient Qi—life-force	Produced from Spleen and Stomach

- Jing is produced when Congenital Qi and Nutrient Qi mix together.

- Protective Qi is produced when Jing mixes with Heavenly Qi from the Lungs.

- Wei Qi, Zhong Qi and Qi are part of the protective Qi life-force energy of the body.

Using facial diagnosis in conjunction with the Five Organs

TCM identifies areas of the face with each of the Five Organs as follows:

1. The forehead represents the Heart.

2. The chin represents the Kidneys.

3. The area under the right eye represents the Lung.

4. The area under the left eye represents the Liver.

5. The area at the tip of the nose represents the Spleen.

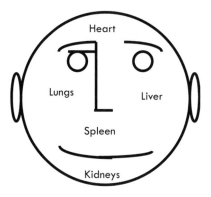

Figure 1.9: Areas of the face

But for our purpose within the 3E Method approach we will use the face as a *whole*.

The five basic sickness conditions in the "whole face" approach

In each of these conditions the face coloration has a different meaning as outlined in Tables 1.6–1.10.

Table 1.6 Sickness of the Heart

Face color	Related element	Prognosis	Explanation
Red	Fire	Normal	Organ color
Black	Water	Bad	Water extinguishes Fire
White	Metal	Bad	Metal overcomes Fire
Green	Wood	Good	Wood produces Fire
Yellow	Earth	Good	Fire produces Earth

Table 1.7 Sickness of the Liver

Face color	Related element	Prognosis	Explanation
Green	Wood	Normal	Organ color
White	Metal	Bad	Metal cuts Wood
Yellow	Earth	Bad	Earth overcomes Wood
Red	Fire	Good	Wood produces Fire
Black	Water	Good	Water produces Wood

Table 1.8 Sickness of the Kidney

Face color	Related element	Prognosis	Explanation
Black	Water	Normal	Organ color
Red	Fire	Bad	Fire overcomes Water
Yellow	Earth	Bad	Earth absorbs Water
Green	Wood	Good	Water produces Wood
White	Metal	Good	Metal produces Water

Table 1.9 Sickness of the Spleen

Face color	Related element	Prognosis	Explanation
Yellow	Earth	Normal	Organ color
Black	Water	Bad	Water overcomes Earth
Green	Wood	Bad	Wood depletes Earth
White	Metal	Good	Earth produces Metal
Red	Fire	Good	Fire produces Earth

Table 1.10 Sickness of the Lung

Face color	Related element	Prognosis	Explanation
White	Metal	Normal	Organ color
Green	Wood	Bad	Wood overcomes Metal
Red	Fire	Bad	Fire melts Metal
Yellow	Earth	Good	Earth produces Metal
Black	Water	Good	Metal produces Water

Face: Color and complexion

"All Qi and blood of all the Meridians flow upwards into the Face." *Nei Jing* (*The Yellow Emperor's Classic of Internal Medicine*)

A person's facial color and complexion will depend on factors such as ethnic or racial origin, occupational, and/or climatic exposure.

HEALTHY FACE

A healthy face glows, and is moist and shiny.

- *In illness*: when the face appears healthy or close to it, it suggests that the Qi and blood are not affected and the illness is not serious.

- *In serious illness*: the face is often lusterless and withered, suggesting depletion of Qi and blood.

THE FIVE COLORATIONS OR DISCOLORATIONS OF THE FACE

1. *White face or pallor:*

   - Bright but puffy indicates deficient Qi/Yang.

   - Lusterless and/or withered indicates deficient blood. (In agonizing pain, the patient may show a pale, white face, usually with perspiration on the body.)

2. *Red face*:

   - Indicates Heat Syndrome, especially of Heart and/or Liver.

3. *Yellow face*:

   - Indicates internal dampness, especially of a weak Spleen.

   - Orange-yellow suggests heat dampness (of Yang jaundice).

   - Pale-yellow suggests cold dampness (of Yin Jaundice).

   - Pale yellow and lusterless may be the "anemic" load of deficient blood.

4. *Bluish face* (or bluish-green face):

   - Suggests stagnation of blood and Qi.

5. *Black face* (or dark):

   - Suggests deficiency, particularly of the Kidney (especially evident under the eyes).

   - Darkened face with a deep, dark-looking complexion may suggest a serious illness which may be difficult to treat.

Pulse diagnosis

Pulse diagnosis is of utmost importance in Traditional Chinese Medicine. It is performed on both hands of the patient.

The palpation is done using three fingers, where the central finger is positioned at the region opposite the styloid process of the radius (the bony ridge behind the palm). The other two fingers are on both sides of the central finger, adjoining it.

The three points are named as follows:

1. *Cun*: the position between Guan and the wrist joint.

2. *Guan*: the position opposite the stylus process of the radius bone.

3. *Chi*: the position proximal to Guan.

Each point corresponds to a different organ, as shown in Table 1.11.

Table 1.11 Diagnostic positions of radial pulse according to Dr. Wan

Position	Right hand	Left hand
Cun	Lung	Heart
Guan	Spleen	Liver
Chi	Kidneys	Kidneys

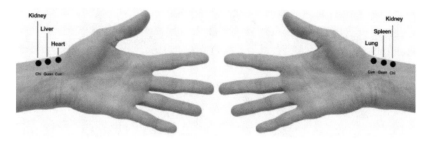

Figure 1.10: Diagnostic positions of radial pulse according to Dr. Wan

The three sections of the body

As illustrated in Figure 1.11 on the following page, the upper burner (Shen Jiao) is from the top of the head to the sternum, the middle burner is from the sternum to the umbilicus, and the lower burner is from the umbilicus to the legs.

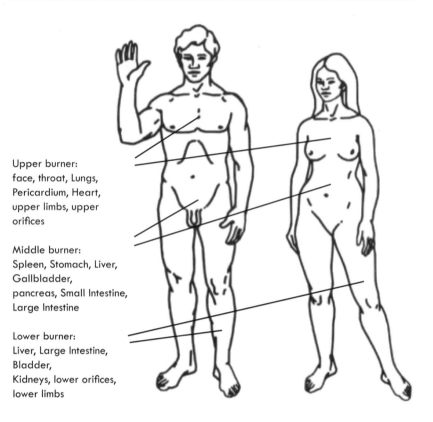

Upper burner:
face, throat, Lungs,
Pericardium, Heart,
upper limbs, upper
orifices

Middle burner:
Spleen, Stomach, Liver,
Gallbladder,
pancreas, Small Intestine,
Large Intestine

Lower burner:
Liver, Large Intestine,
Bladder,
Kidneys, lower orifices,
lower limbs

Figure 1.11: The three sections of the body

Using pulse diagnosis to determine the problem area

The problem area in the body can be found using pulse diagnosis in two ways.

METHOD 1

Place the three fingers lightly on the radial pulse as described earlier. Then determine in which of the fingers the pulse is felt most strongly compared to the other two fingers. Each finger corresponds to a section of the body as follows:

- *Cun*: upper burner.

- *Guan*: middle burner.

- *Chi*: lower burner.

The problem area in the body is determined as follows:

- If strongest pulse is detected in Cun it is the upper burner.

- If strongest pulse is detected in Guan it is the middle burner.

- If strongest pulse is detected in Chi it is the lower burner.

METHOD 2

Place the three fingers lightly as before. Then increase the pressure. Finally increase the pressure even more until you are pressing against the bone. Repeat this until you can determine in which pressure level the pulse was felt the strongest. With this method we do not compare the fingers with each other, but rather the three pressure levels.

The problem area in the body is determined as follows:

- If the strongest pulse is detected using *light* pressure it is the upper burner.

- If the strongest pulse is detected using *medium* pressure it is the middle burner.

- If the strongest pulse is detected using *heavy* pressure it is the lower burner.

COMMENTS

Both methods should be used in order to come to a clear-cut diagnosis.

When asking the patient to describe his or her complaints, the major complaint will usually be mentioned first, within the first few sentences. This information should be compared to the results of the pulse diagnosis. Combining the information from these two sources can in most cases enable the practitioner to identify the major problem section (burner) and organ.

Using the various parameters of the pulse to enhance the diagnosis

The four parameters

1. *Position:* for our purpose in this section we shall use only the superficial (Fou) and deep (Chin) positions. This parameter will help us determine a treatment method (sweating, waiting, or purging using a laxative).

2. *Speed:* normal pulse speed is between 60 and 80 pulses per minute. A pulse below 60 per minute is considered slow. A pulse above 80 per minute is considered fast.

3. *Strength:* we distinguish between strong and weak pulse. Together with pulse rate, the strength of the pulse helps us determine the severity of the sickness and the prognosis as in Table 1.12.

4. *Irregularity:* we distinguish between regular and irregular pulse and/or intermittent pulse. Irregularity in the pulse indicates blood stasis and congestion of the blood.

Table 1.12 Pulses in health and illness according to Dr. Wan

Pulse strength	Healthy person	Sick person
Strong	Indicates strong person	Indicates strong sickness
Weak	Indicates weak person	Indicates weak sickness

According to Table 1.12, in a strong person the pulse would generally feel strong. If a strong sickness attacks the body, the pulse will become stronger as the body's defenses fight back aggressively. If the pulse weakens this means the sickness is not strong.

In a weak person the pulse would generally feel weak. If a strong sickness attacks the body, the pulse will become stronger as the body's defenses fight back aggressively. If the pulse become even weaker this means the sickness is weak.

When the body feels threatened the immune system attacks aggressively, this is seen commonly in most diseases.

Using eye diagnosis in conjunction with the Five Organs

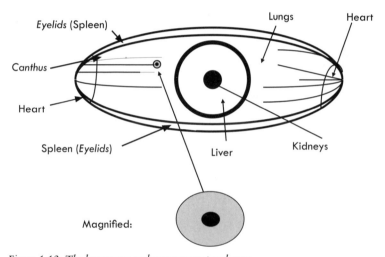

Figure 1.12: The human eye and organ correspondences

Figure 1.12 is a stylized diagram of the human eye. Various parts of the eye represent the Five Organs as follows:

- The top and bottom eyelids represent the Spleen.

- The pupil represents the Kidneys.

- The iris represents the Liver.

- The medial and lateral canthi at both corners of the eye represent the Heart.

- The white of the eye represents the Lungs.

General diagnostic indications

- Pain, swelling = heat, inflammation = excess Fire.

- Itching = allergy = excess Wind.

- Pus, secretion = dampness, infection = excess Water.

Additional signs in the eyes

- Red capillaries represent retention of water in the Stomach.

- Red capillaries reaching the iris represent an allergic condition.

- Dark dots at the end of the capillaries represent blood congestion in the body.

- Grey circles around these dots represent *Chi* congestion.

- Dilated pupils represent Liver and Kidney weakness.

- Changes and discoloration in the iris represent Liver weakness.

- Pink canthi (corners of the eye) represent weak Heart Fire.

- Red canthi represent strong Heart Fire.

- Lumps in whites of the eyes (sclerae) represent scars in the Lungs.

COMMENTS

1. The allergic condition is often related to loss of vitamins, especially B vitamins, which are water soluble and are lost due to water retention in the Stomach.

2. blood congestion, represented by the dark dots (petechiae) in the magnified section of Figure 1.12, indicates older congestion which is more difficult to disperse, while the Qi congestion represented by the grey circles around these dots is newer and easier to disperse.

Using tongue diagnosis in conjunction with the Five Organs

1. Kidneys are represented by the root of the tongue.

2. Liver is represented by the sides of the tongue.

3. Lungs are represented by the tip of the tongue.

4. Heart is represented by the tip of the tongue.

5. Spleen is represented by the remaining area at the center of the tongue.

The healthy tongue and deviations from the norm

First, we must define how a *healthy tongue* looks. If you examine the tongue of a healthy 15-year-old adolescent you will find a good reference point. In general the tongue should be light red, not too red, and not too pale. It should have a fine whitish fur (coating) which is not too moist or thick, and not too dry. It should not be swollen but also not shrunken. When examined it should not tremble or deviate to either side.

Now that we have defined a healthy-looking tongue, we can diagnose illness based on any deviation from the norm, following these guidelines:

47

Seven points

1. *The affected organ* is determined based on the area of the tongue in which an abnormal sign is manifested.

2. *A sore tongue* indicates heat in the corresponding organ. For example, a sore at the tip of the tongue indicates Heart and/or Lung Fire.

3. *No fur* indicates Spleen (digestive) weakness.

4. *No fur accompanied by a thin line* of fur in the center— this line of the tongue is nicknamed "Chicken Heart Fur." This indicates an even weaker Spleen (digestive system).

5. *Thick fur* indicates bad digestion and accumulation of waste matter in the digestive system.

6. *Thick fur at the root of the tongue* indicates a chronic, deep rooted condition.

7. *Teeth marks at the sides of the tongue* indicate water retention in the Stomach.

PAPILLAE

There are three kinds of papillae on the tongue:

1. *The vallate papillae,* which are the biggest; there are approximately 8–12 at the root of the tongue.

2. *The fungiform papillae,* which are smaller and greater in number are dispersed on the sides and the tip.

3. *The filiform papillae,* which are the smallest are also dispersed on the sides and the tip of the tongue.

IMPORTANT POINTS

When there is water retention in the Stomach, resulting in loss of Vitamin B, the papillae protrude and stand out more than in a normal condition. If the depletion of Vitamin B becomes worse the papillae shrink and the tongue surface becomes smooth. If the depletion of Vitamin B worsens further, the papillae shrink even further leaving little holes on the surface of the tongue.

Depletion of Vitamin B can also manifest by a trembling of the tongue when the patient is asked to display the tongue.

The abnormal tongue

The eight tongue body types

1. *Pale tongue* (less red than normal; tinge pink or pale) indicates deficient blood or Qi, or both; or is due to the invasion of exogenous pathogenic cold.

2. *Red tongue* (redder than normal) indicates Heat Syndrome due to either invasion by pathogenic heat (inflammation, infection, of exogenous influence); and/or consumption of Yin (fluid) in various internal organs due to Excess Heat Syndrome.

3. *Scarlet red tongue* (bright red, like a strawberry) indicates excess pathological heat that has penetrated into the deeper internal system of defense (i.e. involving the lymphatic and reticular-lymphatic system).

4. *Purple tongue* (purplish, cyanotic, or bluish-red) indicates stasis or stagnation of Qi and blood flow. A pale purplish tongue suggests stagnation due to Cold Syndrome.

5. *Flabby tongue* (the tongue is larger than normal, flabby, whitish in color, often with teeth imprints in its edges (large, swollen, whitish tongue)) indicates deficiency of Qi and Yang (i.e. a Cold Syndrome) and an internal cold phlegm dampness.

6. *Flabby deep red tongue* indicates possible pathogenic heat in the organs and excess Fire of the Heart.

7. *Crackled tongue* (irregular cracks or cracks on the tongue) indicates general Yin deficiency, i.e. the consumption of body fluids (Yin) by *either* Excess Heat Syndrome and/or in deficient Kidney Yin production, and/or general Yin deficiency.

   Note: a congenital cracked tongue can occur without morbid indications.

8. *Thorny tongue* (red, papillary buds protruding like red spikes on the surface of the tongue) indicates excess pathologic heat, with possible dehydration (deficient Yin).

Tongue mobility

The three types

1. *Rigid and retracted tongue* (tongue is rigid and difficult to protrude, retract or roll around, leading to stuttering) may indicate:

   - invasion of exogenous heat into the body and disturbance of the mind by phlegm

   - heat (Excess Heat Syndrome of Heart)

   - damage of the Liver Yin due to excess heat with the obstruction of the Liver collaterals by wind phlegm (e.g. an alcoholic with Liver impairment).

2. *Trembling tongue* (trembles, wriggles uncontrollably, especially when asked to protrude it) is seen in protracted illness.

- Pale suggests deficient Qi and Yang.

- Red suggests internal wind in organs and meridians.

It can also mean a deficiency in Vitamin B12.

3. *Deviated tongue* (turns to one side on protrusion) indicates obstruction of the meridians and Qi flow by wind phlegm (usually a longstanding diseased condition).

Tongue moss

The five types

1. *Thick moss* indicates "Excess" Syndrome:

   - Pale or pastry moss indicates Excess (Dampness) Cold Syndrome.

   - Thick yellowish moss indicates Excess Heat Syndrome and/or excessive accumulation of food in the Stomach and intestines.

2. *White moss:*

   - Thin pale white moss indicates invasion of the Lung by exogenous wind cold.

   - Thick white moss usually indicates the retention of food (poor digestion due to too much food intake at a time).

   - White sticky moss indicates invasion by exogenous cold dampness and/or retention of phlegm dampness (excessive mucus produced) in the internal organs.

3. *Yellow moss:*

   ■ Thin yellow moss indicates invasion of the Lung by external wind heat.

   ■ Thick yellow moss indicates persistent pathogen, excess food with poor digestion (accumulation of food in the Stomach and intestines).

   ■ Sticky yellow moss (moist) indicates excess damp heat in the internal organs or excess phlegm heat in the Lung.

   ■ Dry yellow moss indicates congestion in the Stomach and intestines (with excess heat and food retention).

4. *Blackish moss* (gray, black):

   ■ Moist blackish moss is seen in Cold Dampness Syndrome, and internal Cold Syndrome of the organs, due to Yang deficiency.

   ■ Dry blackish moss is seen in Yin deficiency due to the consumption by Excess Heat Syndrome of the internal organs.

5. *Peeled moss:*

   ■ Partly peeled, as in geographic tongue in which the surface appearance resembles the geographic outline of a map.

   ■ Total (denuded of moss, a glossy shiny tongue).

   ■ *Both* indicate gross Yin deficiency (with dehydration) especially in a long standing illness where the immune system is tested.

Note: false readings of the tongue may occur, as in:

- the tongue becomes red (redder) with hot beverages

- a grayish black hue or yellowish color coating may be due to food such as certain fruits (plum, olive, oranges, strawberries), colored sweets and such

- smokers and/or drinkers (alcoholic) have a thick yellow moss; strong Darjeeling tea also colors the tongue yellowish-brown.

Stages of sickness and general treatment

Sickness may be defined as:

- the state of being ill

- a particular type of illness or disease

- nausea or vomiting.

Sickness can be classified into three categories:

1. superficial level

2. middle level

3. lower level.

The manifestation of these sickness levels on the tongue is as follows:

- A state of health is manifested in *thin moist white fur.*

- In the early stages, when the sickness is in the superficial level, it is manifested in *thin dry white fur.*

- As the sickness goes deeper into the body and reaches the middle level (Liver, Spleen, intestines) it is manifested in *thin dry yellow fur.*

- As the sickness progresses even further, it goes into the lower level (Liver, Kidneys). This is manifested in *thick dry yellow fur*.

General guidelines for dealing with sickness in the three levels

The following guidelines are based on the principle of assisting the body to heal itself. Following this principle we observe how the body is trying naturally to deal with the disease and assist the body to go in the direction which it has chosen as follows:

- When the sickness is in the upper level we help the body push it out using the *perspiration method*.

- When the sickness is in the middle level we use the *waiting method*. That means that we wait and see whether the body attempts to push the disease out using perspiration or to push it down and out in which case we help it by purging (using laxatives).

- When the sickness is in the lower level we help the body *purge it out* using laxatives.

Note: an extensive description of the above methods can be found in the "Six Syndrome" Model in the Herbal Medicine chapter in this book (Chapter 5).

Six types of bodily constitutions according to Dr. Liew

1. Normal
2. Congestive
3. Phlegmatic
4. Yin deficiency

5. Yang deficiency

6. General weakness, anemic

1. Normal

Good physique, complexion, digestion. Urination and bowel movement normal.

- *Pulse*: strong.

- *Tongue*: little moisture, maybe a little fine whitish fur.

2. Congestive

Dull complexion, lip dark colored, dark under eyelids, epigastrium full.

- *Pulse*: deep and irregular.

- *Tongue*: bluish-purple, purple spots.

3. Phlegmatic

Body stout/rocking, Stomach full-feeling, mouth has sweet and sticky feeling. Body feels heavy, soft stool, mouth dry but patient doesn't like to drink, chest full, dizzy.

- *Pulse*: small regular/slippery.

- *Tongue*: coat wet/sticky.

4. Yin deficiency

Body thin, mouth and throat dry, constipation with internal heat, urine yellow and scanty, thirst cannot be quenched by drinking, insomnia and palpitation, hands and feet warm, loves cold drinks; suffers from tinnitus or deafness.

- *Pulse*: small, stringy and fast.

- *Tongue*: red with little coat or none.

5. Yang deficiency

Pale and stout body, complexion dull, fears cold, lips pale, no taste, extremities cold, stool loose, early morning diarrhea, night urination clear and long, losing hair, suffers from tinnitus or deafness, loves hot drinks.

- *Pulse:* long but weak, soft, slow.

- *Tongue:* pale, swollen, and teeth marks.

6. General weakness, anemic

Pale face, shortness of breath, does not like to talk, weak and dizzy, palpitations and forgetfulness, prolapse of anus, sweats easily under slight exertion, prolapse of uterus, hands numb, menses scanty and pale colored.

- *Pulse:* small and weak.

- *Tongue:* pale colored.

Pulse definitions

- *Small pulse:* only felt in one or two of the positions—Cun, Guan, or Chi.

- *Soft pulse:* feels like a sponge—very little pushback.

- *Long pulse:* the pulse extends past the three positions.

- *Stringy/thin pulse:* the pulse feels like a thin string.

2

RADIAL PULSE

What is pulse? Why is it so important in Chinese medicine?

In the 3E Method we see the pulse as the inner language of the body. The pulse has a flow and specific rhythmic pulsations that have been studied over a long period of time through observation, analysis, and anecdotal recording in Chinese medicine.

Just as external signs and symptoms can be tested so can the pulse be tested with tangible scientific results when done in the correct manner. What needs to be established are the parameters of observation. 3E sets out an *easy*, simple and sound way to study pulse.

A normal radial (Cun Kou) pulse

It is essential to understand that most texts on pulse have been written in Asia using observation of Asian culture, food, and lifestyle. There has not been a significant long-term study on the "normal" pulse in a Western framework, with the many differing ethnicities, cultures, food intake, and lifestyles. We are not going to attempt that here. However, we are going to attempt a "normal" range.

In 3E the features of a "normal" radial (Cun Kou) pulse comprise:

- It would be within the resting pulse rate averages.

- The pulse depth would be *superficial* when felt in the traditional way. The distinction between a superficial and deep pulse is significant.

- When further pressure is applied to the pulse it shouldn't hollow or sink, rather the pulse should fight back, but not too aggressively, as this indicates pathogenesis.

- The consistency of the pulse should not be thin like a fishing line, nor thick like a telephone cable.

- The pulsation of the pulse would be almost vertical and moving towards the thumb.

- The rhythm of the pulse would be regular, steady, and flowing smoothly like a pendulum swing.

- The pulse rhythm and/or beat would not fluctuate between breaths.

Resting pulse rate (RPR)

In 3E the resting pulse rate shouldn't be used in the first or second treatment as an accurate diagnostic tool. An individual's resting pulse rate is discovered over time or over at least 3–5 treatments, not immediately after one session, especially if the patient has an illness.

The best and most accurate way of recording RPR is to ask the patient to record their own pulse on waking in the morning over a period of a few days. This is a great way to get a RPR as when patients come into the office for therapy they may have rushed; it's the middle of the day; after a workout; they are ill, etc. Once the "true" resting pulse is ascertained the practitioner then can use it for proper diagnostic purposes.

But what about RPR in the case of acute illness, for example, influenza? If the practitioner has not seen the patient before, or hasn't any patient history, an accurate RPR would be difficult to ascertain immediately (in fact impossible). Therefore the 3E acupuncturist would take a conservative approach to treatment in this scenario:

Wan's 3E principle: for cold or flu use *shallow* needling. This will ensure that you do not drive the sickness deeper into the body.

Resting pulse rate averages

RPR is subjective to the individual in question. A true resting pulse rate is usually felt in the morning upon waking. In the clinic the practitioner will probably never feel a true resting pulse rate in the patient.

- *Newborn infant 0–1 year:* RPR is usually high, 100–160 beats per minute (bpm). If modern treatments are not working, then needle insertion would appropriately be spot pricking, shallow brief insertions (if at all).

- *Children 1–10 years:* 70–120 bpm. Note that, although a person's immunity is always evolving, it is important to remember that from birth to at least nine years of age a child's fundamental immunity is developing. Treatment would appropriately be aimed at boosting immunity at all times, however in 3E the practitioner will step back a little and let the patient fight the sickness for a short while to help stimulate the immune system before intervention. Usually it is good to wait 24–48 hours before intervention.

- *Children over 10 and adults* (including seniors): 60–100 bpm.

- *Well-trained athletes:* 40–60 bpm.

Pulse regularity

It is imperative to look out for these two types of pulses.

1. Irregular (knotted) pulse

An irregular pulse is like a skipped beat here and there. Like 1, 2, 3, 4/5, 6, 7, 8, 9/10, etc., so it sounds like one, two, three, fourfive, six, seven, eight, nineten, etc. An irregular pulse may be subtle and felt on every 20th or 30th beat, so it needs to be carefully ruled out. Be patient and wait a few minutes when palpating the pulse, to see if there are irregular beats.

An irregular pulse usually signifies a chronic condition and/or blood viscosity. It is easier to treat than an intermittent pulse, however it does represent certain difficulties as it suggests a weakening of the body and blood viscosity.

Always take time to see if your patient has an irregular pulse. An irregular pulse if chronic can progress to intermittent pulse.

2. Intermittent pulse

This pulse is easier to detect than an irregular pulse. The intermittent pulse has an obvious skipped beat pulsation. It also speeds up and slows down at times, sometimes to a gap in between beats. It is especially obvious during inspiration and expiration.

This pulse pertains to Heart problems and represents chronic and hard to treat conditions.

If faced with an intermittent pulse, the road to recovery is difficult—not impossible—just expect a difficult road ahead.

Cross checking

Make sure you compare the left and right radial pulse. Sometimes the left and right side pulses can be different—this is significant.

Pulse depth

Superficial

Most texts state that if a *fast* or *slow* pulse is felt on a superficial position this means exterior pathogens *and/or* the disease is the upper burner, *and/or* it is a superficial (Wei) energy (Qi) problem.

The practitioner would usually add force on palpation to see if the pulse becomes hollow and/or disappears as this signifies a different problem located in deeper immune levels of the body. Of course both problems can co-exist. If the pulse doesn't disappear on heavier palpation but instead *fights back with some force* the problem is usually *in* the upper burner (Heart, Lungs, Pericardium), or exterior (sinus membranes, skin, muscles).

Some examples of superficial pulse signs and symptoms:

- stiff or sore neck

- sore throat

- headache

- toothache (upper)

- sinus pain

- red or painful eyes

- tinnitus

- chest pain, difficulty breathing

- coughing

- fever

- clear thin phlegm, or a light white color

- worry or grief

- sweating

- crying.

Western medicine:

- cold

- influenza

- bronchitis

- pneumonia

- anxiety

- sinusitis

- chronic obstructive pulmonary disease (COPD)

- asthma.

Middle

This pulse depth has several implications. When pressure is applied in feeling the pulse, and the pulse force pushes back more in the middle depth area, this is a "middle depth pulse," but in Wan's 3E we see it as an upper burner problem. Why?

Usually the problem seems to be situated in the middle burner. However, it is not as easy as that. Sometimes the pulse can be suppressed from the upper burner or external pathogenic forces: the superficial energy (Wei) and/or chest (Zhong) energy is failing and the pathogen is heading into the middle burner. Heavenly energy is not being produced effectively in the Lungs thus giving rise to an unhealthy state.

A practitioner needs to consider if the middle depth pulse is the result of failure of Zhong energy or Wei energy in protecting the body. In *Shang Han Lun* (*Treatise on Cold Injury*) by Zhang Zhongjing there are many examples of this issue, such as Taiyang Syndrome progressing to Shaoyang Syndrome.

If the pressure of the pulse is fighting back more forcefully in the middle then the pathogenesis is in the middle burner. However, we still need to treat the chest first. We must get the heavenly energy operating effectively to nourish the body. With middle depth pulse the physician must always assume that there is something wrong in the upper burner, and must take steps to correct this before treating the middle burner.

The illness has been there for a while and is not yet chronic, but soon will be. If the patient feels lethargic with epigastric pain, there is definite Spleen/Stomach involvement.

If the patient feels lethargic with pain under the right hypochondrium, there is definite Liver/Gallbladder involvement.

There can be both Spleen/Stomach and Liver/Gallbladder involvement.

In 3E it is understood that in any chronic cases the Spleen needs to be treated.

It is important to note that when there is middle burner illness the *waiting* method mentioned by Dr. Wan should be implemented, especially if the tongue coating is white/yellow.

Will the body try to sweat, or vomit, or purge the illness?

Some common symptoms of middle burner illness:

- pain in epigastrium

- pain in hypochondrium

- pain in lower abdomen, particularly on right lower quadrant (over cecum area)

- vomiting

- gastric reflux

- chest pain

- frontal and/or temporal and/or vertex headache

- problems with stools, alternating constipation and loose stools

- bloating before and/or during and/or after meals

- lethargy

- pensive (intellectualizing)

- moody (excited then depressed feelings)

- dizzy

- vertigo.

Western medicine:

- irritable bowel syndrome

- Crohn's disease

- ulcerative colitis

- diabetes

- gout

- hepatitis (all kinds)

- gallstones.

It is important to note that even though the pulse is middle level there can still be an ailment in the upper burner, so a middle pulse is usually seen as "sickness in the upper burner." Always be aware of this condition.

Deep

When palpating the pulse, if more force is felt on the deep level of palpation, it is taken as a sign that the pathogen lies in the lower burner at the deep level.

In some texts the deep pulse means the evil energy (illness) has reached the Kidney level or the original (birth) energy. In other texts it is maintained that the Liver is also part of the lower burner and therefore a deep pulse reflects a Liver illness as well as Kidney illness.

In Wan's 3E we see the deep pulse affecting the *entire* body and that *all* organs need strengthening as does the superficial energy, acquired energy, chest energy, fluid (Ying) and blood (Xue) energy. The deep pulse reflects the dwindling of the above forces in the body.

Three organs which should usually be treated in deep pulse conditions: Liver, Spleen, and Kidney. The Kidney needs to be treated because of the location of the pulse, however the Kidney regenerates slowly, much more slowly than do the Liver and Spleen. For this reason the practitioner needs to contemplate a treatment system to deal with this complexity.

A true deep pulse is one of the hardest pulses to treat, especially if accompanied with irregular or intermittent rhythm.

A *good prognosis* is when the pulse has substance and does not fade, and instead fights back a little.

Note: when someone goes into shock the pulse becomes faint, deep, and slows down. If the shock is not treated at once the person can die shortly afterwards, hence:

If the pulse disappears on finger pressure the condition is serious and the life-force is diminished, emergency treatment should ensue.

It is important to note that when the pulse is truly deep, the superficial, chest and general organ energy is diminished, therefore just treating the condition with acupuncture is not enough. Herbal medicine and appropriate supplements need to be given to nourish all the organs of the body with emphasis on the Spleen and Kidneys. With herbal formulas please ensure that the formula prescribed is gentle or low dosage (unless there is a life threatening illness; the patient will most likely be in hospital at this point) for the first few days, then after one week adjust accordingly.

Some common symptoms of deep pulse:

- general weakness
- fatigue
- low libido
- chronic illness—*any* kind
- serious illness—*any* kind
- knee pain
- general aches and pain, ongoing
- diminished concentration levels
- difficulty in breathing
- difficulty in doing anything
- sleeping all the time
- fainting regularly
- much pain
- and many more.

Western medicine:

- any type of wasting disease (e.g. multiple sclerosis)
- menopause
- some forms of cancer
- arthritis—all kinds
- chronic pain
- heart attack

- shock

- weak heart

- and many more.

Pulse characters: Fundamental

The author has encountered many problems in seeking correct pulse positions in the Cun, Guan, and Chi areas. Even old texts are contradictory, so we employ Dr. Wan's model from diagnostics (see Table 1.11 and Figure 1.10, page 41).

Pulse character can be confusing for many reasons. Experience usually makes the practitioner better at diagnosis, after having felt tens of thousands of pulses. When beginning to study the pulse, it remains difficult to identify a "clear" character as there are so many variations.

For example, a slippery pulse. What does a slippery pulse feel like? How is it identified? In the beginning the student depends on text and theoretical descriptions, and a good teacher can show the student what a slippery pulse feels like, however this would take a considerable amount of time. Learning even the minimum 36 pulses is difficult to achieve where only 1000 hours or fewer are spent in clinical study for most practitioners in school.

In 3E importance is placed on diagnosing where the actual problem originates rather than its character. So, as discussed earlier, once the location of the problem has been isolated, the treatment then flows accordingly.

There are over 40 different characteristics of pulse, all representing different problems, and unless you have had experience in feeling all of them at one time or another, it remains a difficult skill to acquire. It comes down to experience and acquired knowledge over time. In the beginning simplification and strong basics is the place to start, with time and experience the character of pulse will be grasped correctly.

Thirteen common pulses

According to Dr. Liew, the 13 common pulses that relate to TCM are as follows:

1. *Hollow*: loss of blood, depletion of essence, depletion of blood, sometimes in males it means ejaculation. It can mean Yin nutrient depletion and anemia.

2. *Tense*: pulling a rope, means cold.

3. *Taut*: middle and lower burner disease, Gallbladder disease, disease of prolonged duration, guitar string.

4. *Soft*: Yang insufficient.

5. *Hollow*: blood insufficient/anemia/bleeding.

6. *Hesitant (spiky/jerky)*: congestion.

7. *Long huge*: body overworking; not much blood in blood vessels.

8. *Short*: sharpness, leading to blood stasis, blockage of Qi and blood.

9. *Swinging*: fullness built up in abdomen, arteriosclerotic, blood is too thick, enriched.

10. *Pearly*: congelation, pregnancy.

11. *Slippery*: oily, water retention, phlegm.

12. *Floating*: superficial, Lung-Taiyang condition.

13. *Thin*: Yin deficiency.

Testing for health

Sometimes patients ask, "Am I healthy? Is my pulse good?"

First, if the patient is not suffering any particular ailment or illness, and is generally in a good state, then the practitioner can test for health using pulse.

A healthy, strong pulse has a substantial amount of "push back" when the practitioner applies a certain amount of force with the three fingers. When applying force on the deep level, a healthy pulse will fight back. This is known as "testing the root."

Note that when someone is ill, a strong push back can indicate a strong illness, e.g. extreme constipation. Usually the test is done when the patient is free from any disease.

Tangible pulse: Result and observation

It is fundamental to establish a *tangible* pulse-result at the beginning, during, and end of each treatment. When an acupuncture point is stimulated so a pulse-result needs to be observed and recorded. How else does a practitioner find out if his/her choice of points and manipulation being used are correct? This step is essential in monitoring the therapy.

In 3E, if the pulse does not fluctuate favorably with the insertion and then manipulation of the needle either immediately or within a few minutes, an unsuitable point has been chosen and/or unsuitable manipulation has been used.

If we use many points at the same time, how do we test which points are having the desired effect? In 3E we usually use one point at a time. Once the diagnosis has been made and channel/point chosen we then insert the needle. Immediate observation and recording of the results follows. If the condition is serious we use two, a maximum of three, points at the same time.

To put it simply, a weak pulse on palpation needs to "feel" stronger on palpation during and after treatment, this equals a "favorable" outcome. A strong bounding pulse needs to "feel" weaker within the treatment time, of course with some conditions it takes longer. However, this does not invalidate the premise that a "favorable" result needs be felt, even if only slight, as may be the case with chronic and/or serious cases.

In 3E if needling does *not* cause a "favorable result" in the pulse the practitioner may be doing one or a few things incorrectly:

- Using unsuitable points or channels.

- Using unsuitable manipulation.

- Diagnosis is incorrect.

- The disease is serious and difficult to treat.

There is a school of practice whereby many points are needled to ensure that if the diagnosis is incorrect the usage of many points will counteract this problem and still provide the patient with a positive result. Wan's 3E regards such an approach as difficult to measure and impossible to assess which points are doing what in the individual.

Summary

In treatment:

- If a pulse is fast make it strive to be slower.

- If a pulse is slow make it strive to be faster.

- If a pulse is deep make it strive for the surface.

- If a pulse is tense/firm make is strive to relax.

- If a pulse is weak make it strive to be stronger.

- If a pulse is strong make it strive to be less strong.

- If a pulse is taut make it strive to become less taut.

- If a pulse is hollow make it strive to fullness.

- If a pulse is full and tight make it strive to be less full and looser.

- If a pulse is slippery make it strive to be steady.

In Chinese medicine, according to Dr. Wan and the *four parameters*:

- If the pulse is strong make it less strong.

- If the pulse is weak make it stronger.

- If the pulse is irregular or intermittent make it regular.

- If the pulse is fast make it slower

- If the pulse is slow make it faster.

Advanced level

When a practitioner has a good level of knowledge and experience of the radial pulse he or she can progress to master level, combining the Ren Ying or carotid pulse in diagnosis and treatment. In this section we will briefly review advanced pulse diagnosis.

The carotid pulse represents the Yang energy of the body. The radial represents the Yin energy of the body (see Huang Fu Mi 2007, Book 2, Chapter 1).

Dr. Wan said that the neck pulse or Ren Ying pulse represents the Yang energy of the body, and the radial pulse or Cun Kou represents the Yin energy or organic energy of the body.

Fundamental I

When palpating both the Ren Ying and Cun Kou, the practitioner should be careful and gentle. Even pressure should be applied to ascertain if the strength of the two different pulses are the same in rhythm and push back pressure.

If they are equal in pressure and strength this represents Yin and Yang harmony.

Fundamental II

If the Ren Ying pulse is stronger, this may indicate a Yang condition and/or a deficient Yin condition.

Fundamental III

If the Cun Kou pulse is stronger, this may indicate a Yin condition, and/or a deficient Yang condition.

3

3E ACUPRESSURE

Introduction

Acupressure is an essential tool and adjunct in acupuncture therapy. It is sometimes underestimated and frequently not used at all. In Wan's 3E Method, however, it is used in nearly every treatment.

The first section of this chapter can be carried out without the guidance of a teacher; it is simple and straightforward. The hand acupressure method techniques require some guidance and a little time to master.

The starting point

Muscle meridians

Acupressure has a great effect on muscle meridians as the life-force energy flows quickly throughout these channels, which are commonly classed as exterior to the body or superficial. Sometimes acupuncture needs a little help breaking through blockages in these channels. Acupressure can assist acupuncture therapy on many levels.

As most of the acupressure points are acupuncture points it is not really necessary to learn about the anatomy and location of muscle meridians as they lie close to their related acupuncture channel. If you are not familiar with the muscle meridians then you will need to learn about them for the acupressure method.

The neurological system in relation to acupressure

The points along the spine are essential in any Acupressure treatment protocol.

In this case it is important to stimulate the Huatojaji points and the Bladder channel line closest to the spine before any tactile therapy. These points also have a direct effect on the central nervous system. When these points are stimulated they excite the nervous system and brainstem in particular. This excitement helps to make the acupuncture treatment more effective.

Huatojaji points in particular are the points chosen in the first method to stimulate the nervous system and thus also excite the brain. The Method in this case is derived from the Japanese acupressure system. Dr. Wan adopted this system using what he called a "presser" but today is known as a "probe." My preference is the "Tsumo-Shin" probe.

Using Tsumo-Shin: Method 1

This system is usually used prior to acupuncture therapy, and it can also be used in conjunction with hand or manual acupressure.

After performing diagnosis while the patient is in the prone position:

- Prepare the spine by using 70 percent isopropyl alcohol and swab both the Huatojaji line and Bladder line closest to the spine until you see red tracks or the blood comes to the surface.

- Locate the points in the Huatojaji channel that correspond with the Shu points. Dr. Wan usually stimulated Bl 11, 13, 15, 17, 18, 19, 21, 23, 25, and Du Mo 3.

- With the Tsumo-Shin tool press these points on both sides of the spine.

- Proceed with acupuncture therapy.

Hand acupressure: Method 2

Method 2 is employed broadly to assist superficial circulation. The Tsumo-Shin method is used to specifically stimulate the nervous system. Acupressure can be applied either alone, or in conjunction with acupuncture therapy.

Usually the Taiyang system responds the most effectively to Method 2 acupressure therapy, then Shaoyang. These two systems give the most effective responses to acupressure as they are closer to the surface. They are also the longest channels in the body externally, and thus exert a strong influence in the four limbs and trunk.

Acupressure techniques

- Press and follow, unblocking the meridian flow.

- Rotating acupressure.

- Isotonic acupressure.

- Therapeutic, from superficial to deep.

- Following bone technique, "chasing the tendon."

- Use the elbow to apply pressure in the hips.

Acupressure points

The points below have been selected to be the most effective in acupressure therapy. The author has observed and tested these points for over 15 years with effective results. The most effective points below are the Taiyang and Shaoyang. The rest can also be used, but the effect is not as fast and dynamic.

TAIYANG

- *Both Bladder lines on the back*: Huatojaji and use the Tsumo-Shin.

75

- *Bl 58 and 59*: all back problems, ankle issues.

- *Bl 36 and 37*: good for unlocking the posterior leg muscles.

- *Si 3*: neck, occipital region, scapula.

SHAOYANG

- *Th 5*: head + aches, ear, upper limbs, upper torso.

- *Gb 34, 39*: lateral parts of the body and legs; helps with any tension.

- *Gb 20, 21*: to help unlock any neck or temporal problems.

- *Gb 30*: for any hip problems.

YANGMING

- *Li 4, 11*: eyes, face, shoulder.

- *St 36, 37, 40*: knees, Stomach, abdomen in general, chest problems.

TAIYIN

- *Sp 6*: calms the mind, lower abdomen pain.

SHAOYIN

Press and follow:

- *Kd 1 mainly*: relaxes mind, good for lower back.

- *Kd 3 and Kd 6 area*: good for tonification.

JUEYIN

Press and follow:

- *Pc 6*: effective with fingernail pressure for nausea, chest oppression, anxiety, worry.

- *Lv 2–3*: good for genital issues, and for calming emotions.

These points are generally not as effective as the others in acupressure therapy.

Treatment zones

Treatment zones are central locations that cover essential areas in the back. These areas come from Dr. Liew's Hannya Massage Therapy teachings.

- *Zone A*: Cervical 6–Thoracic 3. Use Huatojaji points and Bladder Line 1.

- *Zone B*: Lumbar 1–Sacral 1. Use Huatojaji points and Bladder Line 1.

- *Zone C*: Base of Skull. Points Du Mo 16, Bl 10, Gb 20 and Gb 12.

- *Zone D*: Hip–Gb 30 as the center. Reach into both Bladder lines with elbow tip.

Treatment application

Special manipulations in conjunction with acupuncture

- *Kd 3 and Bl 60* at the same time when patient is prone: helps to release the lower back, and relax the mind in stressful cases.

- *Bl 36 and 37* when patient is prone: to release tension in the entire body and also for any back pain.

- *Bl 10* is effective when treating the Bladder channel for neck problems.

- *Gb 20, 21* is very effective when treating the Gallbladder channel for any kind of neck problem and upper limb problem.

■ *Gb 30* with elbow: to unlock the Qi and muscle meridians in the hip prior to acupuncture.

Acupressure in relation to pulse

■ *To slow down a pulse*: use a strong and rigorous manipulation. Treatment should be longer, 45 minutes or more.

■ *To speed up a pulse*: use slow and direct manipulation (holding). Treatment should be shorter, 30 minutes or less.

■ *When a pulse is weak*: less is better, with slow application (usually no longer than 25 minutes).

■ *When a pulse is strong* (sickness is strong): release zone A, B, C, D—apply acupressure on both Bladder lines on back (usually take 45–50 minutes).

■ *When a pulse is deep*: always use gentle pressure with slow application. Treatment should be 30 minutes or less.

■ *To regulate a pulse* when confused with pulse reading: Apply general therapy (see "Relaxation and general treatment" on the following page).

Treatment protocols

Trauma and accidents

After corrective procedure (life support, surgery, for instance) has taken place, the life-force of the body will try to establish itself. In the event of surgery or major changes (fractures, organ transplants, etc.) the life-force may have difficulty finding its way.

There may be major blockages of channels and the practitioner should use gentle application for the first few treatments and the treatment time should generally be no longer than 25 minutes. As the practitioner sees improvement then more rigorous, deeper, or stronger application can follow.

Injuries and illness

- Depending on area of injury or illness, unlock Zone A, B, C, or D.

- Apply appropriate points (as stated above) using isotonic (constant) pressure with strong or not so strong force as discussed above.

- Use the Ahshi method (also known as De-Qi, "obtains Qi"), stimulate points where there is pain—this always works well.

Relaxation and general treatment

- Unlock Zones A, B, C, and D.

- Usually bombard both Bladder lines on the back with circulating acupressure, from superficial to deep, 3–4 times for each line.

- Stimulate Bl points 36 and 37 using press and follow technique.

- Stimulate Kd 3 and Bl 60 at the same time with thumb and index.

- Stimulate Du Mo 20–24 (press and follow technique).

Golden rule: always feel pulse before, during, and after treatment.

General rule: if the acupressure therapy fails to work in the muscle meridians it usually means:

1. wrong diagnosis and or therapy

2. it is beyond acupressure—the disease or complaint is rooted in deeper body systems.

4

3E ACUPUNCTURE:
THE ESSENTIALS

Introduction

This chapter provides the foundation of Wan's 3E Method of acupuncture treatment. If the reader does not have access to a teacher then read this chapter, apply the 3E Method, and re-read.

To gain maximum effectiveness the practitioner needs to apply this section repeatedly, and refer to it over a number of years. The information seems at first basic and easy; however, the knowledge is hard to come by in such a concise format.

It is also important to try not to mix other philosophies or methods; just stick to what follows here, apply the 3E Method, and then test the effects and monitor the results.

The Verses

The five domains

DOMAIN 1: DISEASE, ILLNESS, OR SYNDROMES OF ANY KIND, SYSTEMIC

Use *one* point in each meridian at a time unless the condition is severe and needs very powerful sedation. (I never witnessed Dr. Wan using more than one point in a channel at a time, unless he applied Vitamin B12 injection therapy and/or the fire needle method, or "opening the channel" method.)

3E ACUPUNCTURE: THE ESSENTIALS

The most effective acupuncture points lie below the elbow on the arms and below the knee on the legs.

- Use one leg point when general = [+].

- Use two points when ill, one arm and one leg = [++].

- Use three points (or more), one arm, one leg, and one or more back points, bleeding technique or moxa, when the sickness is serious = [+++].

Explanation
Before we choose points we need to assess the severity of the problem at hand. This system is a matter of simplifying and making it *easy* to write notes.

1. +: the patient does not have a serious problem and is not ill, or has a minor complaint, needs better general health or perhaps preventive management.

2. ++: the patient is ill, low grade fever, common cold, digestive problems, etc.

3. +++: the patient is seriously ill, high fever, stroke, sciatica, deficiency patterns, etc.

4. ++++: the patient is chronically ill, the disease is long standing, elderly (over 70), has weak constitution, *strong* acute condition, post partum, post operative, etc.

For a weak, debilitated patient, enduring illness, *strong* acute illness, elderly (over 70) use:

- Shu, Huatojaji, and Du Mo points *prior* to using arm and leg points.

- Ren channel can be used prior to or after using arm and leg points = [++++].

Always treat the Yang channel (brother) before using Yin channel (sister). For example, if we want to treat the Lung we should treat the Large Intestine first. If we want to treat the Liver, we should treat the Gallbladder channel first. Not doing so may drive the illness deeper. This is also referred to as "treating the hollow before the solid."

When treating Li 11, St 36 to 40, Gb 34 to 39 the limbs should be bent.

DOMAIN 2: ACUPUNCTURE MANIPULATION

Dr. Wan stated that only tonification and sedation is used in acupuncture manipulation. Dr. Wan Le Ting stated that:

> Logically there is no such thing as "neither vacuity nor repletion," for if there is neither vacuity nor repletion, then Yin and Yang are in balance and this condition does not require acupuncture treatment. Therefore in hand technique there should be no such thing as even supplementing/even drainage. To supplement is to supplement. To drain is to drain.

DOMAIN 3: PAIN, INJURIES, AND PARALYSIS

For arm and leg injuries: use the healthy limb, on the opposite side to the injured limb, in acupuncture for pain, injuries and especially paralysis. Always treat the better side, for example, if there is pain in the left elbow use Li 11 on the right elbow. This is known as "opposite side therapy."

For body injuries: one can treat the site of injury with fire needle and/or moxa application above the surface of the affected area and/or 3E spot pricking method to the area of injury prior to acupuncture therapy on the opposite side of the body.

Dr. Wang Le Ting stated: "In hemiplegia, while administering the operation clinically, first puncture the healthy side and later the affected side to supplement the righteous Qi and to dispel the evil Qi, this is what is meant by guiding the Qi and blood to support immobility and wilting" (see Hui Chan Yu and Ru Han Fu 1999, p.56).

The *Shi Er Xue Zhu Za Bing Ge* (The *Rhyme of the Twelve Points Ruling the Miscellaneous Diseases*) states (of Li 11 and Gb 34): "When using them in clinic, if there is one-sided upper limb or lower limb joint pain, first select the healthy side" (Hui Chan Yu and Fu Ru Han p.59).

For any type of back injury: if appropriate[1] use Wan's 3E spot pricking method or fire needle and/or moxa on site of injury, then use distal acupuncture point on opposite side/ healthy side.

If not appropriate use distal acupuncture point, for example for injury to L2 or L3 area use Bl 40 or Bl 60 on opposite side of affected area.

For acute injuries on limbs: if appropriate[1] use Wan's 3E spot pricking method or fire needle and/or moxa on injured area, then sedate the corresponding or appropriate point on the opposite side.

If not appropriate sedate using corresponding or appropriate point on the opposite side of affected area. For example, if right lateral knee pain, sedate Gb 34 on left leg.

DOMAIN 4: GENERAL WEAKNESS, EXHAUSTION, ELDERLY, AND PROLONGED ILLNESS

For all general weakness and prolonged illness: employ Ren 4 with or without moxa in every treatment, usually after the chosen treatment.

For people over 70 years of age with a slow pulse: use Ren 4 and St 36 as a general rule, with sedation–tonification method and/or moxa after the chosen treatment.

When the pulse is deep and/or the condition does not go away with acupuncture or moxa: use herbal medicine to assist the acupuncture method.

With any patient with weak constitution and/or prolonged illness, if wanting to apply tonification to a point: sedate the point on insertion by twisting the needle anti-clockwise during the insertion. Keep sedating after insertion for a brief period, using a minimum of 9 thrusts to a maximum of 36 thrusts, then apply tonification, starting with 9–18 thrusts with clockwise twist. This is known in 3E as the *sedation–tonification method.*

DOMAIN 5: DIFFICULT ISSUES—THE OBSCURE CONDITIONS

For breakdown of the whole body with cold limbs (total Yang collapse): use Ren 8 with moxa with salt and ginger technique. (Monitor the salt carefully as it can burn the patient.)

Spot pricking Well points of the hand in addition to acupuncture is very effective for *emotional disorders, heat patterns,* and *acute disorders.*

When confronted with a *serious condition* and the practitioner is unclear about the problem at hand employ the balance Yin and Yang method.[2] Spot prick all Well points of the hand and then Daidun (Du Mo) 26.

For fever: always employ Du Mo 14 with sedation method prior to using other acupuncture points. Spot pricking can be applied on Huatojaji and/or Shut points prior to acupuncture. If the patient is in a convulsive state: spot prick all hand Well points first, then use Du Mo 14 prior to using other acupuncture points.[3]

To lift energy or for the *collapse of Yang,* e.g. prolapsed syndrome or similar: tonify Du Mo 20 along with other points. If the patient has Cold Syndrome use moxa on this point as well.

---

1   That is, if the condition is Excess Heat use bleeding method prior to using acupuncture. If deficient or cold, use fire needle or moxa prior to and/or after using acupuncture.

2   In clinical practice we are sometimes confronted with serious illness and nothing seems to make sense in diagnostics. Sometimes our knowledge is not sufficient to deal with the issue at hand. Of course these days we can simply refer to the hospital. But if confronted use the balance Yin and Yang method. This technique can also be used for patients in a coma state.

3   Nowadays patients in this condition are more likely to be admitted to hospital.

Manipulation preference

Manipulation preference is shown in Table 4.1. There are many other techniques in Traditional Chinese Medicine: a good source of knowledge is *A Study of Daoist Acupuncture and Moxibustion* (see Cheng Tsai Liu, Lui Zheng Cai and Ka Hua 1999). We can use other forms of manipulation learned elsewhere if we wish to enhance the effect.

Table 4.1 Tonification and sedation

Tonification	Sedation
Insertion: End of breathing out	End of breathing in
Withdrawal: End of breathing in	End of breathing out
*3 forceful thrusts *in*: 1 slow/gentle thrust *out*	**1 slow/gentle thrust *in*: 3 forceful thrusts *out*
Slightly *clockwise* rotation	Anti-clockwise (120–180 degrees)
Rx	
To supplement	To sedate
For *general* treatment 5–12 minutes with constant stimulation every 3 minutes	For *general* treatment 15–25 minutes with constant stimulation every 3 minutes. Use heavy stimulation for serious cases
Gentle tonification: 3–21 thrusts (total in one session) Aggressive tonification: 21–45+ thrusts (total in one session)	Gentle sedation: 9–27 thrusts (total in one session) Aggressive sedation: 27–54+ thrusts (total in one session)

Note: the general rule with any insertion is to always start from the superficial (epidermis) level first then work the needle deeper if necessary.
Key:
* always start the first jab as superficial, then middle, then deep thrust action. Then slow thrust *out*.
** before plunging deep, attain the De-Qi first. Then deep thrust, middle thrust, superficial thrust. Then *in*.

Needle insertion and manipulation for body types

BIGGER BODY TYPES OR OVERWEIGHT TYPES

Attain the De-Qi on insertion then insert needle to *deep* level and *retain* for longer than usual.

NORMAL OR THIN BODY TYPES

Shallow insertion, retain needle; subject to pulse fluctuation—the life-force energy will fluctuate quicker than the bigger body type.

Channel selection

Table 4.2 outlines which side to use when selecting a meridian and point according to Dr. Wan. There is a similarity with Dr. Wang Le Ting on this issue on energetic focus, but there is a difference in terms of point selection. Dr. Wang Le Ting, and most other texts, suggest needling bilaterally. Dr. Wan insists on using one point in each meridian at a time; in this the 3E Method is unique.

As Dr. Wang Le Ting states: "Yang Qi descends and is down borne. Yin Qi rises and is up borne. The Left up bears and the Right down bears" (Hui Chan Yu and Fu Ru Han, p.23). The Yang flows down the right side and the Yin flows up the left side. Choose points and channels from the tables below.

Table 4.2 Channel selection

Lung:	Use right side	*Large Intestine:*	Use right side
Spleen:	Use right side	*Stomach:*	Use right side
Heart:	Use left side	*Small Intestine:*	Use left side
Kidney:	Neutral	*Bladder:*	Neutral
Pericardium:	Use left side	*Triple burner:*	Neutral
Liver:	Use left side	*Gallbladder:*	Use right side

Table 4.3 The most commonly-used points in acupuncture according to Dr. Wan

Channel	Most effective points
Lung	Lu 7 and 9
Large Intestine	Li 4 and 11
Stomach	St 36 and 40, 42
Spleen	Sp 6 and 3
Heart	Ht 6 and 7
Small Intestine	Si 3
Bladder	Bl 40, 60 and 62
Kidney	Kd 3 and 6
Pericardium	Pc 6
Triple burner	Th 5
Gallbladder	Gb 34 and 41 usually with sedation
Liver	Lv 2 and 3
Du Mo	Du Mo 4, 14, and 20
Ren	Ren 3, 4, 6, and 12
Well points of hand	Using spot prick method

Acupuncture insertion and retention according to pulse

The practitioner should use Table 4.1 for guidance on needle manipulation and Table 4.2 for guidance on selecting channels *for all types* of pulse.

Table 4.4 refers to *insertion and withdrawal* of acupuncture needles in relation to common pulse types. With experience and consistent results, the practitioner will eventually come to an understanding of the Method. Please remember that the information comes from many years of practice.

Table 4.4 Insertion, depth, retention, and withdrawal of ten common pulses according to Dr. Liew

Pulse	Insertion	Depth	Retention	Withdrawal
Fast	Quick	Deep	Long retention	Slow
Slow	Quick	Shallow	Short retention	Quick
Deep	Slow	Deep	Short retention	Quick
Deep and slow	Quick	Deep	Short retention	Quick
Deep and fast	Slow	Deep	Long retention	Slow
Thin	Quick	Shallow	Short retention	Quick
Large	Quick	Shallow	Short retention	Quick
Slippery	Quick	Shallow	Depends on pulse	Quick
Rough/jerky	Massage above point before	Shallow	Short retention	Massage below point after
Pearly/hesitant	Massage above point before	Shallow	Short retention	Massage below point after

Note:
Large pulse: felt beyond the three positions.
Thin pulse: hard to feel, like a thin piece of string.
Slippery: oily feeling, slips away from the fingers, moves away upon pressure.

Manipulation for syndromes

HEAT SYNDROME

Cooling manipulation, spot prick Bl 40, 3E bleeding method (needs to be shown by teacher).

COLD SYNDROME

Use heat manipulation and moxa.

- *Cooling manipulation:* involves using sedation at all three levels of depth.

- *heat manipulation*: involves using tonification at all three levels of depth.

The Eight Extraordinary Vessels

These channels are important in treatment for conditions that do not respond when employing acupuncture on the 14 main meridians. When the points of the 14 main meridians are not getting the required effect, a practitioner needs to consider using the points on the eight extra channels. A practitioner with experience can sense when the points of the 14 main meridians are not having the intended effect, in this case it is a good idea to consider using the connecting points of the eight extra meridians.

Gatherings from Eminent Acupuncturists (*Zhen Jiu Ju Ying*) states: "This treatment method [i.e. the method of using the opening and coupled points of an Extraordinary Vessel] is very broad indeed. It is known as setting a very broad net in open country to catch a single rabbit." This means to catch the rabbit (in this case, illness) in a huge field (the body). We can also certainly use the points in times of knowing as well, and they are very effective points indeed. The quotation refers to the state of trying to catch something difficult or elusive in a vast area.

> When disease and illness are elusive employ the points of the Eight Extraordinary Vessels.

The point selections in Table 4.5 are the connecting points of the Eight Extraordinary Vessels. *These are the points of choice in the 3E Method.*

Table 4.5 The Eight Extraordinary Vessels: Connecting points

Control point	Meridians
"Broken sequence" **Lu 7**	**Ren** chest, throat, Lung
"Shining sea" **Kd 6**	**Yinqiao** chest, throat, Lung
"Back stream" **Si 3**	**Du Mo** inner canthus, neck, shoulder, back
"Ninth channel" **Bl 62**	**Yangqiao** inner canthus, neck, shoulder, back
"Inner gate" **Pc 6**	**Yinwei** Heart, chest, Stomach
"Minute connecting channels" **Sp 4**	**Chong** Heart, chest, Stomach
"Outer gate" **Th 5**	**Yangwei** auricular, outer canthus, cheek
"Falling tears" **Gb 41**	**Dai (belt)** inguinal area, hip, menstrual area, eyes, neck

The points are paired as Table 4.4 suggests:

- Lu 7 with Kd 6
- Si 3 with Bl 62
- Pc 6 with Sp 4
- Th 5 with Gb 41.

When to use arm or leg or both? Please refer to Domain 3 in the Verses (page 82).

Putting it all together: Getting started

The five considerations

How do we tie all the information above together? This simple case study shows how to locate points after a diagnosis.

A 27-year-old male patient suffers from recent coughing with little phlegm. He is also suffering from slight chest pain but his condition does not stop him from carrying out his daily duties. His pulse is superficial and fast. His tongue has a white coating.

The diagnosis is wind cold invasion in the Taiyang. What channels and points are appropriate using the 3E Method?

1. *What is the severity of the condition?*
   According to the Verses, Domain 1 (page 80), this patient may have a [+] problem.

   Explanation: recent cough and fast, superficial pulse but he can carry out daily duties. It sounds like a minor complaint.

2. *Which channel or channels are appropriate?*
   According to the diagnostics the problem is in the *Taiyang*. For [+] sickness we are going to use the leg channel = *Bladder*.

3. *Which point or points are appropriate?*
   According to the Verses, Domain 1, for [+] sickness we should use *one Leg point below the knee.*

   According to Table 4.3 we have three points to choose from. Bl 62 is an excellent point for wind cold (author's choice).

4. *Which side should we use the point on?*
   According to Table 4.2, Bladder is neutral. This means we can use the point on either side. As this is more of a Yang problem, the right side is chosen.

5. *Whether to tonify or sedate?*
   In this case the pulse is fast and superficial. The patient is not deficient, so it is a [+] diagnosis. Therefore the pulse should be *slowed down.*

   According to Table 4.1, the sedation method should be employed.

Solution: the result after using the five considerations is *Bl 62, the right leg* with the *sedation method*.

If the result is not favorable, i.e. the pulse does not fluctuate towards a healthy state after the sedation method has been applied to Bl 62, the practitioner can employ an arm point. (In this case Si 3 with the sedation method.) In the above case it is not a serious condition so these two points should be more than sufficient.

Important notes
WHEN TO USE SHU POINTS

Domain 1 of the Verses states: a chronic condition, long standing illness, elderly (over 70) and strong acute illness is classified as a [++++] problem (page 81).

After the diagnosis of a [++++] problem, the patient should be directed to lie in the prone position. After application of Tsumo-shin acupressure, the practitioner can proceed to use Huatojaji or Shu points and/or other back points of choice.

In using the Shu points one point is classified as using both sides of the spine. So, in other words, if treating Bl 15 both sides will be treated and counted as one point.

In treating the Shu we generally use 1–3 points at the same time, 4–5 for more serious conditions. Time of needling should be no longer than 15–20 minutes. In the 3E Method, the sedation–tonification method in Domain 4 (page 83) of the Verses is the usual stimulation employed for cases of deficiency and weakness.

SPECIFIC TECHNIQUE FOR [++++] ILLNESSES USING ARM OR LEG POINTS

If the practitioner intends to use the tonification technique in any [++++] condition it is advisable to use the sedation–tonification method (Domain 4, page 83) prior to tonification.

After applying the sedation technique check to see if the pulses are fluctuating favorably. If they are, stick with the sedation.

If sedation is not effective, quickly change the stimulation to tonification. This will ensure that the disease will not be driven into deeper levels of the body energy.

COMMON POINTS

If the common points shown in Table 4.3 do not bring about the intended result, then the practitioner should feel free to use other points. Table 4.3 is included as a guide to Dr. Wan's most frequently used points, this does not imply that other points are not effective.

"Open the channels" method

For long channels such as the Bladder and Gallbladder channels, sometimes it is good to "open up" the channel by using gentle sedation on points such as Bladder 10 or Gallbladder 20 before conducting main treatment. The Bladder and Gallbladder channels are long and winding and often get blocked easily; sometimes we need to add more stimulation in the upper part for the lower part to unblock and vice versa.

A few doctors insist on using Gb 20 points even before diagnosis, as they feel this "opens up" the energy flow to the brain, and therefore should be employed before any other therapy or treatment.

In the 3E Method we use this "opening up" if we are not achieving the intended results.

FOR NECK, UPPER TORSO, AND UPPER LIMBS

Sedate (gently or aggressively) either Gb 20, or Bl 10 for 5–10 minutes prior to performing arm or leg acupuncture. (Gently in this case means 9–27 sedative thrusts. Aggressive is 27–54 sedative thrusts, really aggressive is 54+ sedative thrusts, as per Table 4.1.)

FOR HIP, LOWER BACK, AND LOWER LIMBS

■ For hip, sedate (gently or aggressively, see above) Gb 30 for 5–10 mins whilst patient is prone prior to using Gb 34.

■ For lower back or lower limb problems, sedate (gently or aggressively) 5–10 minutes or spot prick Bl 40 whilst patient is prone *prior* to using Bl 60 in supine position.

In this case we are using two points in one channel; however, they are not implemented at the same time.

Caution and rules

Some rules are meant to be broken, but *not these two*!

1. *Rule 1*: do not use sedation on more than three Yang points per treatment. This is the maximum number of points per treatment. Spot pricking can be employed along with the maximum three points.

2. *Rule 2*: do not sedate more than one Yin point per treatment. In 3E we usually do not sedate Yin other than the Lung channel.

If a patient has a Yang collapse or severe Yang deficiency, employ tonification and/or moxa on Yang points first such as Du Mo 4, 14, and 20 before using sedation on any Yin points. It is extremely rare to see an exuberant Yin condition. (The author has *never* seen this condition.)

Serious conditions with exuberant Yang

This includes conditions with a body temperature of more than 100 degrees Fahrenheit (40 degrees Celsius); severe steaming bone disorders, heat stroke, etc.

THE FIVE METHODS TO ARREST YANG WITH ACUPUNCTURE

1. Employ 3E bleeding technique to *all* (meaning the five Zang organ Shu points and diaphragm Bl 17) *or* appropriate Shu points in conjunction with spot pricking Bladder 40.

2. Then using the sedation method employ Du Mo 14 with aggressive manipulation; retain for longer than usual (27–54+ thrusts).

If 1 and 2 do not yield a sufficient result then the condition is serious, and the following points should be added:

3. *For less serious cases*: employ one Yang arm point first, then, when finished, employ one Yang leg point (use Li 4 and St 42). When completed spot prick appropriate Well points on the right hand (e.g. Lu 11 for sore throat). Use aggressive sedation (54+) on both points.

4. *For more serious cases*: employ one Yang arm point first, then, after a few minutes, employ one Yang leg point (use Li 4 and St 42). Retain both points at the same time. When completed spot prick appropriate Well points on the right hand. Use aggressive to really aggressive sedation (54+) on both points.

5. *For really serious cases*: employ both Yang points of arm and leg at the same time and retain for 45–60 minutes (use Li 4 and St 42). When completed spot prick all Well points on both hands. Use really aggressive sedation (108+).

If the above is insufficient and does not arrest the condition especially after employing point 5 call the ambulance service immediately.

3E HERBAL MEDICINE: COLD AND HOT SYNDROMES

Introduction

The aim of this chapter is to highlight the differences between current modern TCM and the 3E Method with regard to the "Six Syndrome" Model of *Shang Han Lun,* and the four stages of Warm Disease Theory. The philosophy and science is clarified between these differing views to give insight into the 3E Method.

Custom prescriptions

Once the practitioner has mastered the understanding of the syndromes, it will be easy to prescribe custom formulas. It is important to understand the mechanisms of diagnostics discussed in Chapter 1 before prescribing custom formulations, which are learnt over time. The knowledge in this chapter gives the practitioner strong foundations in the understanding of how herbal medicine is used in the 3E Method. Once the principle is understood, custom preparations become simple and easy to prescribe.

The eight classifications of herbal formula actions

1. *Nutritive:* for prevention and strengthening.

2. *Tonic:* to excite, to boost.

3. *Perspiration*: for upper burner issues.

4. *Purging*: to send pathogens down (or help the body to send pathogens down).

5. *Harmonizing*.

6. *Clearing*: for skin diseases, abscess, carbuncles, etc.

7. *Heating*.

8. *Cooling*.

Fundamentals

For cooking

Herbs are used in cooking on a daily basis to invigorate life-force energy and strengthen blood, bones, general health, etc. This use is nothing unusual; herbs such as Shan Yao, Gou Gi Zhi, Dang Gui, Da Zao, ginger, turmeric, etc. are used in many countries on a daily basis.

The method of preparation is somewhat different in daily cooking. As cooking is generally directed by flavor, herbal medicine is directed by extracting therapeutic properties. So whilst cooking, herbal properties can be utilized for health, but the extraction method is the most effective therapeutically.

In sickness

In the 3E Method acupuncture is usually applied first in therapy prior to using herbs. Chinese herbal medicine is usually used when and/or if:

■ the disease is longstanding, for example, a cold that does not go away

■ chronic disease

■ the pulse is deep with whatever character

- for patients with weak or deficient constitutions
- for patients over the age of 70 in general
- for patients with malnutrition
- for patients who are exhausted, and have been weak for a prolonged period
- postpartum
- post-operative
- for the syndromes hot, cold, and damp.

Preventive

Herbs can also be used as a preventative to sickness. A formula such as Xue Fu Zhu Yu Tang for moving blood, for example, is taken daily for helping the blood circulation. Chinese medicine, in sum, however, is much more than just taking herbal medicine and getting acupuncture. Practitioners should not forget the other ingredients in preventive therapy:

- daily meditation
- chanting
- gentle exercise
- correct nutrition
- healthy lifestyle
- minimizing the taxations
- social charity.

Tonics

Herbal medicines can be used as tonics for all kinds of issues, such as cooling the body, improving immune function, boosting libido, increasing energy, etc.

Caution: do not give tonics to a patient suffering from any long-term illness, or serious illness. When the body is deficient and exhausted, treatment focus should be on *nourishing* not boosting. Boosting with tonics may exhaust the patient and drive the sickness in further, and/or give strength to the disease, thus making it stronger. Hence the rule: do not give Huang Qi to patients with cancer.

Vital nutrition

Usually in modern countries food hygiene is high and the food standard reasonable. Nutrition issues like malnutrition in countries such as Australia, the U.S., and Europe are not as common as in countries such as Africa and India.

Instead, in Australia, the U.S., and other Western countries, people suffer from indulgence or "too much of a good thing," like ingesting too much fried food, alcohol, candy, soda, fast food, etc. In general the nutrition quality is better in these countries but healthy eating practices are not always followed. We also have the problem of genetically modified food which has been shown to be detrimental to health (see Smith 2007).

The body is dependent on good nutrition. Herbal medicine is like an essential source of nutrition.

Herbal medicines can be seen as an organic nutrients in essence. They give the organs of the body direct essence in the form of nutrition and also energy, whether it be hot, cold, warm, or cool energy. It is energy whose character differs from the therapy of acupuncture.

In the 3E Method herbal medicine is seen as organic nutrition that helps sustain the life-force of the body, thus facilitating correct harmony and function. Acupuncture is a therapy that helps to regulate the life-force of the energetic body when in disharmony. But without nutrients there is no physical body.

Efficiency and economics

In the 3E Method we always emphasize efficiency and economics. The questions are always: What will work the most effectively for the condition at hand? What is also the most cost-effective means? Usually acupuncture works fast because it is hands-on, tactile therapy. Herbal medicine requires more effort in dispensation, and takes longer to feel the effects. Sometimes for certain deficiency patterns a patient may need to take a herbal mixture for months.

Review of diagnostics: Stages of sickness and general treatment

This is intended to refresh understanding of the stages of sickness in relation to herbal medicine.

Sickness can be classified into three categories:

1. superficial level

2. middle level

3. lower level.

The manifestation of these sickness levels on the tongue is as follows:

- A state of health is manifested in *thin moist white fur.*

- At the early stages, when the sickness is in the superficial level, it is manifested in *thin dry white fur.*

- As the sickness goes deeper into the body and reaches the middle level (Liver, Spleen, intestines) it is manifested in *thin dry yellow fur.*

- As the sickness progresses even further, it goes into the lower level (Liver, Kidneys). This is manifested in *thick dry yellow fur.*

General guidelines for dealing with sickness in the three levels

The following guidelines are based on the principle of *assisting the body to heal itself.* Following this principle we observe how the body is trying naturally to deal with the disease and we assist the body to go in the direction which it has chosen, as follows:

- When the sickness is in the upper level we help the body push it out using the *perspiration method.*

- When the sickness is in the middle level we use the *waiting method.* That means that we wait and see whether the body attempts to push the disease out using perspiration or to push it down and out by purging (using laxatives).

- When the sickness is in the lower level we help the body *purge it* out using laxatives.

Making a diagnosis using the Six Syndrome Model

The "Six Syndrome" Diagnostic Model is a condensed method based on the Meridians and Collaterals Theory. It is used mainly for dealing with diseases caused by exogenous pathological forces. This model includes six syndromes which have to be memorized and recognized.

Each of the syndromes is related to specific meridians and organs in the body. Also, each of the syndromes represents a condition of sickness which sums up the following factors:

- the level of penetration or progression of the attacking pathogenic energy or force

- the meridians and organs that are affected

- the strength of the defending (antipathogenic force) energy of the body.

Each syndrome has a recommended treatment strategy, so once we identify the syndrome, we automatically have general guidelines for treatment.

Diseases caused by exogenous pathogenic factors usually penetrate the body and progress from the outside, through the middle to the inside, but there are exceptions. The progression of the disease is often manifested in the way the syndromes evolve. We will shortly list them in their natural order of evolution.

The syndromes are grouped into two groups: Yang Syndromes and Yin Syndromes.

The Yang Syndromes

All the Yang Syndromes are characterized by the following:

■ strong antipathogenic energy of the body (defending Qi, resistance)

■ hyperactive pathogenic factor

■ active disease condition

■ heat and excess symptoms.

The general treatment strategy for the Yang Syndromes is to eliminate the pathogenic factor and the excess heat.

Table 5.1 The Yang Syndromes' main individual characteristics

Syndrome	Aspect	Meridian/ organ	Main symptoms
Taiyang	Back	Bl, Si	Neck rigid, pain in back of head and neck
Shaoyang	Side	Gb, Th	Fullness and distension in costal and hypochondriac regions
Yangming	Front	Li, St	Flushed face, abdominal pain, and fullness

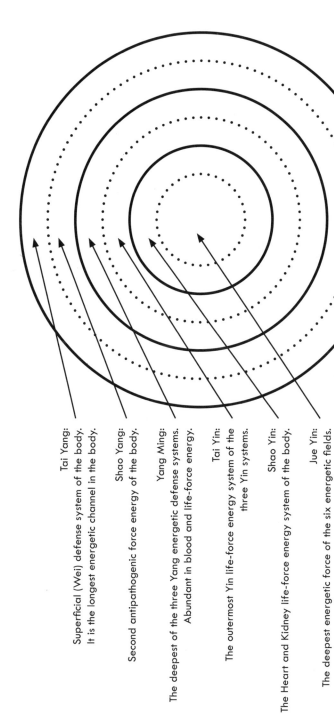

Tai Yang:
Superficial (Wei) defense system of the body.
It is the longest energetic channel in the body.

Shao Yang:
Second antipathogenic force energy of the body.

Yang Ming:
The deepest of the three Yang energetic defense systems.
Abundant in blood and life-force energy.

Tai Yin:
The outermost Yin life-force energy system of the
three Yin systems.

Shao Yin:
The Heart and Kidney life-force energy system of the body.

Jue Yin:
The deepest energetic force of the six energetic fields.

Figure 5.1: The six energy systems of the body

1. INITIAL YANG SYNDROME (TAI YANG BING)

Location: the fight between the external pathogenic energetic force and the body's defending energetic force (Wei Qi) is at the exterior, close to the surface.

Disease stage: often at the initial stage of a disease caused by an invasion of a disease caused by an exogenous factor.

General symptoms: fever, aversion to cold, stiffness, and pain of the back of the head and neck; superficial pulse. When Bladder is affected (Taiyang Fu organ) water retention and dysuria may result.

Variations

1. Taiyang caused by an invasion of wind results in sweating and slow or slowing superficial pulse.

2. Taiyang caused by an invasion of cold results in no sweating and tense pulse.

3. Taiyang Fu Syndrome caused by invading pathogen leading to retention of water in the Bladder.

Treatment: help the body *push out* the external pathogenic force. Restabilize energetic force circulation in the Taiyang meridians.

Analysis

Type I—febrile disease caused by wind.

Specific symptoms: fever, sore throat, perspiration, chill

Pulse: superficial, fast or slow, tense

Tongue: tip of tongue red, white coat or little coat

Formula: Gui Zhi Tang. Stiff neck add Ge gen. Profuse phlegm add Fu ling.

Type II—febrile disease caused by cold.

Specific symptoms: with or without fever, but with chill and pain in the body, nausea, vomiting, and pulse tense both in Yin and Yang. *No perspiration.*

Pulse: tense, superficial.

Tongue: pale, white coating.

Formula: Ma Huang Tang + additions (if needed).

Type III—wWater retention leading to inability of fluids to stream upward (as restriction of Yang Qi). Tai Yang Fu Syndrome.

Explanation: invading pathogen leading to retention of water in the Bladder. External pathogen remaining in the exterior of the body. Pathogen may be of wind or wind heat.

Specific symptoms: difficulty in or dribbling urination, lower abdominal distension, dysfunction of the Bladder in opening and closing. Thirst but with vomiting immediately after drinking. Chills and fever, headache.

Pulse: floating, may be rapid.

Tongue: red tip, white or white yellow thin coat, moist.

Formula: Wu ling San.

2. LESSER YANG SYNDROME (SHAO YANG BING)

Location: the pathogenic factor has penetrated deeper into the mid section of the body.

Disease stage: Shaoyang is a progression of Taiyang. Shaoyang is an intermediate stage between Taiyang and Yangming.

Meaning of symptoms: the external pathogenic factor which has penetrated the body's mid section is resisted by defensive Qi there. This battle creates alternating fever and chills. It also results in disturbance of Qi flow in the middle level. Rising Stomach Qi creates anorexia and vomiting. Rising Gallbladder Qi creates a bitter taste in the mouth, dryness of the throat, and blurred vision. Rising Qi disturbs the mind.

Treatment: harmonize the Shaoyang meridians and organs and strengthen the body. *Use the waiting method.* Once the body gathers enough force it will push the pathogenic factor outwards either by sweating or downwards by purging.

Analysis

Symptoms: alternating fever and chills. Fullness in the costal and hypochondriac regions, dizziness, anorexia, mental restlessness, deafness, vomiting, bitter taste in the mouth, dryness of throat, and blurred vision.

Pulse: taut, rapid, slender, middle, wiry.

Tongue: mix yellow/white, greasy coat.

Formula: Xiao Chai Hu Tang + additions.

Please note: although we are using the waiting method, Xiao Chai Hu Tang is a formula that works on harmonizing the middle burner. Harmonizing can be used to help strengthen the body so it can carry out its natural action.

3. GREATER YANG SYNDROME (YANG MING BING)

Location: deep level. Inside the body interior.

Disease stage: Yangming is a progression of Shaoyang. The pathogenic factor has penetrated the interior of the body, resulting in a very strong fight between the external pathogenic factor and the body's resisting antipathogenic force. This creates excessive heat inside the body. The heat consumes body fluids.

Variations

1. Yangming Meridian Syndrome, where the heat spreads all over the body.

2. Yangming Fu Organ Syndrome, where the heat accumulates in related Fu organs.

3.1 Yangming Meridian Syndrome

Symptoms: high fever, profuse sweating, extreme thirst, flushed face, mental restlessness.

Meaning of symptoms: the pathogenic factor has invaded the Yangming meridian. The strong resistance creates strong endogenous heat. The heat manifests in high fever and flushed face. The heat expels body fluids causing profuse sweating. The heat consumes body fluids. These cause extreme thirst and dry yellow tongue coating. The heat also rises and disrupts the mind resulting in restlessness and irritability. The strong battle between the external pathogenic force and the body's defensive antipathogenic force coupled with the high heat causes a strong and superficial pulse.

Treatment: clearing the excess heat using the purgation method.

Analysis

Stomach excess of pathogenic factor.

Exterior Syndrome: fever, spontaneous perspiration with fear of heat, but no fear of cold, thirsty.

Pulse: long, fast, rolling, superficial, and forceful.

Tongue: dry yellow coat.

Formula: Bai Hu Tang with additions—in *Shang Han Lun.*

In the 3E Method we use *Gui Zhi Tang Jia* (with) *Shi Gao* 15–20 gm and *Zhi Mu* 5–8 gm.

3.2 Yangming Fu Organ Syndrome

Symptoms: fever which is aggravated in the afternoon, abdominal fullness and pain which is aggravated by pressure, constipation, restlessness, delirium.

Meaning of symptoms: the heat in the Yangming Fu Organ (Stomach and Large Intestine) moving downwards dries the faeces and creates constipation, fullness, and pain aggravated by pressure and a deep forceful pulse. The Yangming meridian is at its peak activity in the afternoon. That superimposes on the fever condition resulting from the sickness, creating a rise in the fever during the afternoon. Excessive heat rising upwards disturbs the mind and creates a dry yellow tongue coating as described earlier.

Treatment: the purging method is used to clear excess heat.

Analysis

Tidal Fever with high grade heat is excess condition—Tidal Fever with low grade heat is due to Yin deficiency or damp heat.

3.3 Fu Syndrome (Interior)

Symptoms: fever which is aggravated in the afternoon, abdominal fullness and pain which is aggravated by pressure, constipation, restlessness, delirium.

Pulse: deep, forceful, excessive type pulse.

Tongue: dry yellow tongue coating or burnt yellow tongue coating with thorns on the tongue.

Formula: Da Cheng Qi Tang.

The Yin Syndromes

All the Yin Syndromes are characterized by the following:

- weak antipathogenic force of the body (defending Qi, resistance)

- hyperactive pathogenic factor

- inactive disease condition

- cold and deficiency symptoms.

The general treatment strategy for the Yin Syndromes is to strengthen the defensive antipathogenic force energy and nourish the body.

Table 5.2 The Yin Syndromes' main individual characteristics

Syndrome	Meridian/organ	Main symptoms
Taiyin	Lu, Sp	Abdominal pain and diarrhea
Shaoyin	Ki, Ht	Dryness of mouth and throat
Jueyin	Li, Per	Pain and heat sensation in the Heart; pain at top of the head

1. INITIAL YIN SYNDROME (TAI YIN BING)

Cold deficiency type syndrome with retention of internal dampness resulting mainly from constitutional deficiency of Spleen Qi and/or invasion of external pathogenic cold.

Symptoms: abdominal fullness, abdominal pain alleviated by pressure and application of heat, vomiting, poor appetite, diarrhea, no thirst, prolapsed uterus or anus.

Meaning of symptoms: deficient Spleen Qi results in poor transporting and transforming of fluids leading to retention of internal cold dampness. This results in lack of thirst, diarrhea, pale tongue, and white tongue coating. Deficient

Yang in the middle burner results in abnormal flow of Qi from the middle burner, both upwards and downwards. This results in vomiting, poor appetite, abdominal fullness, abdominal pain.

Treatment: warming up the middle burner. Dispersing cold dampness.

Analysis

Pulse: deep, slow or slowing pulse.

Tongue: pale with white coating.

Formula: *Si Jun Zi Tang*, or *Li Jun Zi Tang* or *Ren Shen Tang*.

2. LESSER YIN SYNDROME (SHAO YIN BING)

This syndrome represents a condition of systemic weakness, mainly of the Heart and Kidneys due to pathological changes which have taken place in these organs. In such a condition, the body's defensive antipathogenic force energy is very weak.

Variations

The systemic weakness represented by the Shaoyin Syndrome can lead to two variations:

1. The Cold Shaoyin Syndrome, where deficient Yang leaves Yin unchecked, and coupled with pathogenic factors creates a Cold Syndrome.

2. The Heat Shaoyin Syndrome, where deficient Yin leaves Yang unchecked, and coupled with pathogenic factors creates a Heat Syndrome.

2.1 The Cold Shaoyin Syndrome

Symptoms: aversion to cold. Lying in a curled position. Desire to sleep. Apathy. Cold limbs. Diarrhea with undigested food. No thirst. Preference for hot drinks. Profuse clear urine.

Meaning of symptoms: this syndrome is often a result of deficient Heart and Kidney Yang coupled by an exogenic pathogenic cold. Not enough heat is generated to warm the body. This creates cold limbs, an aversion to cold, apathy, and sleepiness. This also affects Spleen Yang resulting in diarrhea with undigested food and profuse clear urine. This Cold Syndrome also results in preference for hot drinks and lack of thirst unless the diarrhea and/or deficient transportation of body fluids creates a condition where not enough fluids reach the upper part of the body, resulting in thirst.

Treatment: nourish the Yang and warm to eliminate the cold.

Analysis

Two types in cold:

1. Heart Yang deficiency leading to poor promotion of mind. The patient has a tendency to fall asleep, intolerance to cold, aversion to cold, and coldness of the four limbs.

2. Yang deficiency in Spleen and Kidney. The more severe type will show watery diarrhea with undigested food or dawn diarrhea, chills, and curls themselves in bed with coldness at the extremities.

Pulse: deep, slow, weak, minute/thready.

Tongue: pale, white coat, puffy, delicate.

Formula: *Si Ni Tang*—the older the sickness the less the *Fu Zi*.

2.2 The Heat Shaoyin Syndrome

Symptoms: restlessness, insomnia, dryness of mouth and throat, deep-yellow urine.

Meaning of symptoms: this syndrome can be a result of two conditions: (1) constitutional deficiency of Kidney Yin coupled with an invasion of an exogenous pathogenic heat leading to a Heat Syndrome; (2) consumption of Kidney Yin by persistent pathogenic heat. Deficient Kidney Yin results in hyperactive Heart Fire, causing restlessness and insomnia. Consumption of Kidney Yin by heat creates thirst and dryness of throat and mouth, a red or deep-red tongue. heat and hyperactive Heart Fire causes a rapid thready pulse.

Treatment: nourish the Yin. Clear the heat.

Analysis

Two types in heat:

1. Heart and Kidney Yin deficiency. Deficient heat flaring up stirring the mind, insomnia, irritability, vexation.

2. Deficiency heat steaming body fluids out. Deficiency heat consuming body fluids. Night sweats, dry mouth and throat.

Pulse: deep thin/thready and rapid.

Tongue: red or deep red.

Formula: *Huang Lian e Jiao Tang*.

3. GREATER YIN SYNDROME (JUE YIN BING)

This syndrome represents a condition where body Yin has almost been totally depleted. The Yin–Yang balance has been severely disrupted. The body's defensive antipathogenic force energy has been depleted. It is a complex Cold–Heat Syndrome.

Symptoms: emaciation, thirst, hunger with no desire to eat, cold limbs, diarrhea, vomiting or vomiting of roundworms. Hot painful sensation in the chest. A feeling of rising flow in the chest.

Meaning of symptoms: a complex Cold–Heat Syndrome gives rise to complex symptoms: depletion of Yin and consumption of body fluids creates thirst and emaciation. Hyperactive Liver Yang causes hunger, yet cold deficient Stomach and intestines result in no appetite. Abnormal flow of Yang energy prevents it from reaching the limbs, resulting in cold limbs. Abnormal upward flow of Yang heat creates a painful hot sensation and feeling of upward flow in the chest. Disturbance of energy force flow in Stomach and intestines results in diarrhea and vomiting.

Treatment: warming the cold organs and at the same time clearing the heat. Nourishing and reinforcement of Yin and at the same time elimination of heat.

Analysis

Yang collapse:

Symptoms: total exhaustion of Yang. Always sleeping. Great thirst with frequent urination, an uncomfortable feeling of ascending air rushing up from below the epigastrium, a hot and painful feeling in the chest, or the Stomach, and hunger without being able to take in food. Once food is taken, ascarids will be vomited up. If a purgative is given, there will be continuous diarrhea.

Pulse: deep, slow, tense, even cannot be felt.

Tongue: pale, teeth marks, swollen.

Formula: *Fu Zi Jia Gui Zhi Tang*. For worms add *Wu Mei Tang*. *Wu Mei Tang* should be given mid morning before the patient has something to eat.

Preventive

When the cold weather arrives it is good to have patients take a pre-emptive approach to illness. In the 3E Method the formula of choice is *Gui Zhi Tang*. Taking this formula in between seasons helps to strengthen the body immune system. Why? Particularly at the end of summer, there may be latent damp or damp/heat pathogens lingering in the body. It is a good idea to strengthen the immunity and remove these lingering pathogens (if any) prior to the cold season, otherwise they can linger and cause illness. If there are no lingering pathogens, it is still a good idea to strengthen and nourish the body to prepare for the cold season ahead.

Gui Zhi Tang

Gui Zhi	Cinnamon twig	10 gm
Bai Shao	White peony root	10 gm
Sheng Jiang	Ginger (raw)	10 gm
Da Zao	Chinese black date	5 pieces
Zhi Gan Cao	Stir fried with honey licorice root	6 gm

Note: *Gui Zhi Tang* can be taken twice a week to help keep the Wei, Qi and Ying energy well nourished. In most texts the dosage is usually lower, in the 3E Method we use 10 gm as the baseline for most herbs and we usually add 6 gm of *Zhi Gan Cao* instead of 3 gm.

Other methods for prevention

- Using moxa at Guan Yuan, Ren 4, for 10–15 minutes daily for about 15–30 days at the junction of summer and autumn. This helps to foster a stronger constitution and helps the body push out any latent or lingering pathogens from late summer heat.

- Gentle Qi building exercises, 15–20 mins a day.

- Daily meditation.

- Eating healthily.

- Avoiding stress.

Warm diseases

Diseases in a warm or hot external environment have a different effect on the body from diseases caused by cold. One of the two major differences is the lingering of damp and/or damp/heat pathogens and the problems associated with them. The other is the invasion of noxious heat and Fire pathogens that can consume body fluid rapidly. The 3E Method is in agreement with much of standard Chinese medical theory when it comes to the Ying and Xue levels. Where there is disparity is the Wei and Qi levels, which will be discussed below.

The four levels

According to Maciocia (2000) the four levels of warm disease are as follows:

1. Defensive Qi level (Wei level):

- wind heat

- damp heat

- summer heat

- wind dry heat

2. Qi level:

- Lung heat

- Stomach heat

- Stomach and intestines dry heat

- Gallbladder heat

- Stomach and Spleen damp heat

3. Nutritive Qi level:

- heat in Pericardium

- heat in Nutritive Qi

4. Blood level:

- heat victorious agitates blood

- heat victorious stirs wind

- empty wind agitates in the interior

- collapse of Yin

- collapse of Yang

General summary
WEI FEN ZHENG WEI (SUPERFICIAL DEFENSIVE) LEVEL SYNDROME

Syndrome of the Wei (superficial defensive) system.

Explanation: early stage of a febrile disease when only the superficial part of the defensive life-force energy is involved.

Symptoms: fever and chilliness, headache, general aching, hypohidrosis.

Tongue: whitish fur of the tongue.

Pulse: floating and rapid pulse, etc.

QI FEN ZHENG QI (SECONDARY DEFENSIVE) LEVEL SYNDROME

Syndrome of the Qi (secondary defensive) system.

Explanation: the second stage of a febrile disease with the channels of the Lung, Gallbladder, Spleen, Stomach, or Large Intestine being involved.

Symptoms: high fever, sweats, dire thirst, flushed face, scanty urine, constipation.

Tongue: yellow coat of the tongue.

Pulse: rapid, slippery, or gigantic.

YING FEN ZHENG YING (NUTRIENT) LEVEL SYNDROME

Syndrome of the Ying (nutrient) system.

Explanation: serious development of a febrile disease with involvement of the central nervous system: brain, spinal cord, meninges, etc. Body fluid being consumed in the Pericardium and Liver affecting consciousness.

Symptoms: high fever, restlessness, insomnia, delirium, or even loss of consciousness in severe cases.

Tongue: deep red body.

Pulse: thin/fine, rapid.

XUE FEN ZHENG XUE (BLOOD) LEVEL SYNDROME

Syndrome of the Xue (blood) system.

Explanation: high fever, febrile disease at its severest stage, characterized by severe damage of vital essence and blood, with various forms of bleeding such as hemoptysis, epistaxis, hematuria, in addition to high fever, coma, etc.

Tongue: dark red body, may have cracks, may be thorny.

Pulse: thin, racing, deep.

Superficial level Syndromes

As mentioned previously the focus of the 3E Herbal Method is to support the body to carry out its function. In this case we have:

- the perspiration method
- the waiting method
- the purging method.

The 3E Method differs from Wu Jutang's theory in the Wei level Syndrome in terms of herbal formula choice. Remembering that the body maintains body temperature for homeostasis at 98.6 degrees Fahrenheit (37 degrees Celsius), the external environment and external pathogens can alter this homeostasis at any time. Our job is to help the body maintain homeostasis as much as possible, keeping in mind that the body's natural defense against disease may be to raise temperature as in the case of fever which acts as a natural antibiotic by inhibiting replication of pathogenic bacteria.

EXPLANATION OF WEI LEVEL SYNDROME DUE TO WARM DISEASES

If the heat, wind, damp, or Fire pathogen is able to enter the body, this condition usually means that the Wei or Qi level is deficient, and/or the pathogen is extremely strong.

In whichever case the Wei, Qi, and Ying levels need support to carry out their duty. Even in summer or late summer the body's natural reaction to external pathogens is to heat up. In the case of deficient Wei (defensive) Qi, we need to help the body *push the illness out* and normalize the defensive energy using the *perspiration* method. In the case of the pathogen overpowering a healthy immune system we still need to help the body clear the pathogen with the perspiration method.

In *Yin Qiao San* there are few if any herbs to support the Wei, Qi, and Ying level, however Yin Qiao San does attack the pathogen. We need to remember that the body's antipathogenic life-force immunity is supported by nutrition, heat, and energy, and when the body's antipathogenic life-force energy is under attack it needs help to flourish both from a nutritive level and energetic level. "When the righteous Qi recovers, then the disease symptoms are automatically cured, this is what is meant by the principle of supporting the righteous and dispelling evils" (Hui Chan Yu and Fu Ru Han 1997, p.69).

Analysis

Two main formulas are used for Wei level Syndrome by Wu Jutang: *Yin Qiao San* and *Sang Ju Yin*.

Yin Qiao San

Jin Yin Hua	Honeysuckle flower
Lian Qiao	Forsythia fruit
Jie Geng	Root of the balloon flower, platycodon
Niu Bang Zi	Great Burdock fruit
Bo He	Field mint
Dan Dou Chi	Prepared soy bean
Jing Jie	Schizonepeta stem
Dan Zhu Ye	Bland bamboo leaves
Xian Lu Gen	Reed rhizome
Gan Cao	Licorice root

When we analyze the above decoction we can see that all the herbs are cold, cool, mild, and/or neutral. The actions of the majority of the herbs are to "clear" heat, and get rid of toxin. There are no herbs to transport essential nutrition to the body's antipathogenic life-force energy to *assist the body to push* the pathogen out. *Yin*

Qiao San has a strong diaphoretic action, and very little effect on nutrient support.

In 3E Method the emphasis is always to nourish the body's antipathogenic life-force energy (Wei, Qi, Ying, and Xue) to support, protect, and augment the life-force so it can carry out its functions. At the same time the external pathogen, whether heat, damp, Fire, or wind, needs to be treated as well.

Sang Ju Yin

Sang Ye	White mulberry leaf
Ju Hua	Chrysanthemum flower
Lian Qiao	Forsythia fruit
Bo He	Field mint
Jie Geng	Root of the balloon flower, platycodon
Xing Ren	Apricot kernel
Lu Gen	Reed rhizome
Gan Cao	Licorice root

Once again in the above formula all the herbs are cold, cool, mild and neutral. They are aimed at diaphoresis and stopping the cough. There are no herbs in this formula that focus on transporting essential nutrition to the body's antipathogenic life-force energy (except *Gan Cao*). The goal is to support and assist the body in carrying out its natural immune function and dispersing the external pathogen.

3E METHOD FOR WEI LEVEL SYNDROMES

We will choose the *perspiration* method because the external pathogen or syndrome is on the surface because the tongue coating is usually white.

Explanation: Wei Syndrome caused by external wind, heat, damp, and Fire.

Symptoms: fever and chilliness, headache, general aching, hypohidrosis, sweating or no sweating.

Tongue: white coating, dry, thin, thick, or moist. Red tip of tongue.

Pulse: superficial/floating, fast or moderate.

Gui Zhi Tang is implemented as the base formula, with additions. For no sweating use *Ma Haung Tang* or add *Ma Huang* to *Gui Zhi Tang*.

Analysis of Gui Zhi decoction

Following is a brief analysis of the energetic component of each herb in the *Gui Zhi* decoction:

Gui Zhi	Cinnamon twig
Bai Shao	White peony root
Sheng Jiang	Ginger (fresh)
Da Zao	Black Chinese date
Zhi Gan Cao	Licorice root stir baked in honey

Gui Zhi

Gui Zhi is warm in nature, attributive to Heart, Lung and Urinary Bladder channel. Heart and Lung in this case refers to Zhong Qi, and Urinary Bladder channel refers to Wei Qi. Induce sweating to expel the exogenous evils from the body surface, for common cold of the wind cold type (see author's note on the following page).

Bai Shao

Slightly cold in nature, attributive to Liver channel. Nourishes blood and astringes Yin. Used for night sweating due to Yin deficiency and spontaneous perspiration due to low body resistance and imbalance between Ying energy and Wei energy. Can also be used for convulsion of Wind Syndrome resulting from sthenic Liver Yang, severe heat, Yin deficiency or blood deficiency.

Sheng Jiang

Slightly warm in nature, attributive to Lung and Spleen channels (protects Taiyin). Induce sweating to expel the exogenous evils from the body surface. For common cold of the wind cold type.

Da Zao

Warm in nature, attributive to Spleen and Stomach channels. Nourish blood and calm the mind. This is an essential herb, in any illness the acquired Qi needs to have a free flow for the body to receive essential nutrition. *Da Zao* facilitates this process effectively. "In treatment the Stomach is first. If a person is diseased and one does not treat the Stomach, on what can they rely for life?" (Hui Chan Yu and Fu Ru Han 1997, p.41).

Zhi Gan Cao

Mild in nature, attributive to Spleen and Stomach channels. Clears away heat and toxic material. In the 3E Method we usually use 6 gm instead of the usual 3 gm. *Zhi Gan Cao* also has the effect of relieving a cough and removing phlegm.

Author's note

Even though *Gui Zhi* and ginger are used in wind cold, we need to clarify an often missed point. In summer or late summer it can be hot or damp, and then there are, at times, *spikes*, where atmospheric temperature drops or rises. It rains, and temperature lowers, or it cools down suddenly; this effect can be seen as wind/cold in summer. For example, when going to the beach on a hot day, the wind turns, and one feels chill, and the body cools down depending on its upright energy to keep homeostasis at 98.6 degrees Fahrenheit. The heat pathogens from the atmosphere try to invade the body as the drop in temperature has compromised the antipathogenic life-force energy.

Analysis

In the brief description of the single herbs above we can see that *Gui Zhi* decoction not only helps to dispel pathogens whether heat, hot, or cold with the perspiration method but also helps to protect and nourish the Wei, Qi, Ying, and a little of the Xue (blood) levels. It also has the effect of arresting a cough.

Gui Zhi Tang is warming and helps the body's antipathogenic life-force energy to flourish, and does not have an exuberant Yang-like action. Therefore it is correct to say that *Gui Zhi Tang* is not a hot formula. The body needs help to keep homeostasis and the temperature at 98.6 degrees Fahrenheit regardless of external environment fluctuations; *Gui Zhi Tang* assists the body to carry out this process.

Additions to *Gui Zhi* decoction for Wei Syndromes

Some examples of herbs to add to the *Gui Zhi* decoction in Wei level Syndromes:

- For external pathogen, heat or Fire: *Niu Bang Zhi, Jin Yin Hua, Lian Qiao,* and to expel external pathogen.

- For phlegm and damp/heat: *Jin Yin Hua, Yi Yi Ren, Niu Bang Zhi, Fu Ling, Jie Geng* for phlegm and dampness.

- For wind/heat: *Fang Feng, Jin Yin Hua, Lian Qiao, Niu Bang Zhi.*

■ For cough: *Xing Ren, Sang Ye, Sang Bai Pi.*

CONCLUSION

In 3E Herbal Method for Wei (superficial) diseases caused by a warm environment *Gui Zhi* decoction is the first formula of choice, with additions. If there is absence of sweating we use *Ma Huang Tang.*

We can add as many toxic clearing, heat clearing, damp removing, wind removing herbs as we wish as long as there is also emphasis on supporting the Wei, Qi, Ying, and Xue systems of the body. Thus the body can carry out its natural function of *perspiration* and pushing out the pathogen.

Qi level Syndromes

In the Qi level there are three common basic tongue coatings:

1. moist/greasy white and/or yellow

2. thin dry yellow

3. thick yellow.

These tongue body types are:

■ red

■ crimson

■ pale

■ pinkish

■ cracks

■ thorny.

The main pulses are:

- rapid

- large

- full

- deep and forceful.

THE WAITING METHOD

Moist/greasy tongue coating

A moist and/or greasy tongue with a thin white coat usually means that the pathogenic dampness has not bound with the Qi dynamic (immune system such as white blood cells surrounding the invader and neutralizing it). Therefore the purgation method should not be employed. When the tongue coat is thin white or white/yellow, and moist or greasy, we usually apply the waiting method.

A moist or greasy tongue means that damp pathogens are abundant in the body, and may be lingering. Use the *waiting method* to see what the body does. The body will usually either try to perspire and push pathogens out, or will try to purge the damp pathogens out. In *Warm Disease Theory* (Wen and Seifert 2000, pp.87–88), Wu Jutang suggests three methods:

1. *Diffusing Qi and transforming dampness* clears the Qi dynamic and damp pathogens during the initial stage of damp warmth. Symptoms of fever during the afternoon, sweating that fails to eliminate fever, mild aversion to cold, oppression in the chest, scant urine, slimy white tongue moss, and soggy, moderate pulse. Its paradigmatic formula is Three Kernels Decoction (*San Ren Tang*).

2. *Discharging heat and drying dampness* uses acrid-opening, bitter-descending combinations to dry dampness and discharge heat when damp warmth becomes trapped and concealed in the middle burner, causing symptoms such as fever, thirst, abdominal distention, nausea, and slimy

125

yellow tongue moss. Its paradigmatic formula is Wang's Coptis and Magnolia Bark Beverage (*Wang Shu Lian Po Yin*).

3. *Scattering damp pathogens* uses bland drying medicinals that generate urine and drain dampness to eliminate pathogens. It is generally prescribed when lower burner blockages cause symptoms such as scant urine, sensations of heat steaming up to the head with subjective feelings of head distention, white tongue moss, and thirst. Its paradigmatic formula is Poria Skin Decoction (*Fu Ling Pi Tang*).

There are circumstances where each of these three methods may be prescribed individually; in practice they are generally used in various combinations. The Qi-diffusing, dampness-transforming method is, for example, normally combined with the dampness-scattering method; whereas the dampness-drying, heat-discharging method is generally used with the Qi-diffusing, dampness-transforming method. Dampness-dispelling methods are also commonly combined with heat-clearing methods, yellowness-abating methods, Stomach-harmonizing methods, and coursing and dispelling methods according to the clinical condition.

When considering the use of the dampness-dispelling method consider whether dampness has already transformed into dryness. If so, dampness-dispelling methods are contraindicated. Likewise, when a patient's Yin fluids are insufficient, the dampness-dispelling method should only be used with caution.

Note that Wu Jutang also used other methods for moist tongue coating. In 3E we use the waiting method. When a disease is neither internally nor externally bound, it is conceptualized as Shaoyang or lesser Yang:

- tongue coating is *moist*, usually white and yellow combined

- tongue body is usually red, or becoming reddened

- pulse is usually wiry/rapid.

The harmonizing and resolving method

Whenever warm disease pathogens are neither externally nor internally bound—when confined in lesser Yang, lodged in the triple burner, or concealed, the harmonizing and resolving method can be used to thrust out pathogenic heat and to diffuse and clear the Qi dynamic. "Harmonizing" is one of the eight major treatment methods and has harmonizing-resolving and coursing-discharging functions to resolve the exterior and harmonize the interior. Its various subdivisions are shown below, according to Wen and Seifert (2000, p.85).

1. *Clearing and discharging lesser Yang* is used primarily to clear and discharge half-external, half-internal lesser Yang pathogenic heat. It can also be used to transform phlegm and harmonize the Stomach. However, its principal application is for heat confined in lesser Yang when there is deficit of the harmonizing and descending functions of the Stomach. It can be used in the presence of symptoms such as alternating fevers and chills, bitter taste in the mouth, rib-side pain, strong thirst, dark yellow urine, Stomach dilations, nausea, slimy yellow tongue moss, red tongue, and string-like rapid pulse. Its paradigmatic formula is Sweet Wormwood and Scutellaria Gallbladder-Clearing Decoction (*Hao Qin Qing Dan Tang*).

2. *Scattering, dispersing, penetrating, and discharging* is used to disperse triple burner Qi aspect pathogens by diffusing the Qi dynamic, and by discharging and transforming phlegm-heat. It is generally administered when pathogens lodge in the triple burner; thus, the failure of Qi transformation leads to turbid phlegm obstruction. Symptoms may appear, such as undulating fevers and chills, chest dilations, abdominal distention, scant urine, and slimy tongue moss. Its paradigmatic prescription is Gallbladder-Warming Decoction (*Wen Dan Tang*). However, commonly-used

medicinal combinations include apricot kernel (*Xing Ren*), magnolia bark (*Hou Po*), and poria (*Fu Ling*).

3. *Membrane source opening and extending* causes turbid, damp pathogens to be disinhibited, coursed, and thrust out. It is used primarily for turbid damp heat confined and blocking the Qi in cases where there are more chills than fever, Stomach dilations, abdominal distention, slimy white tongue moss (like powder piled on the tongue), and crimson tongue. Formulas such as Lei's Membrane Source Diffusing and Outthrusting Method (*Lei Shu Xuan Tou Mo Yuan Fa*) are generally used.

The harmonizing and resolving method is generally combined with other methods, such as the heat-clearing, dampness-transforming method, or the Gallbladder-disinhibiting, yellowness-abating method, as appropriate to the clinical condition.

When considering the use of this method, the following cautions must be observed:

1. While the *lesser Yang clearing and discharging* method can thrust out pathogens and discharge heat, its heat-clearing function is not very strong, and is inadequate when patients have strong internal heat.

2. The *scattering, dispersing, penetrating, and discharging*, and the *membrane source opening and extending* methods are both more effective than the *lesser Yang clearing and discharging* method at coursing and transforming turbid dampness, but they cannot be used when heat is half external and half internal (Wen and Seifert 2000, p.85).

3E Method for moist/greasy tongue

In the 3E Herbal Method, when the tongue is moist/greasy with white or white/yellow (mixed) fur, the waiting method is usually employed. Acupuncture is employed to help the body dispel and discharge heat and toxin, relax and strengthen the bodily processes so they can carry out their function. For herbal medicine it remains unclear whether to use perspiration or purgation so it is better to wait a brief amount of time, normally 24–72 hours. The patient is advised to abstain from cold drinks, raw and/or cold foods, dairy products, sweets, greasy/fried foods, alcohol, caffeine, drugs, and eating late at night, as these factors precipitate lingering dampnes, usually signified by a moist/greasy tongue coating.

Usually when the above method is implemented the body will try to perspire or purge itself. If, after 72 hours, the body is neither perspiring nor purging (thick yellow tongue, deep forceful pulse) this can mean that the life-force energy (Qi dynamic) has not yet been bound with the pathogens. If the patient is not getting weaker or worse in terms of symptoms a further 24–48 hours are allowed to observe whether the body finally finds it way. If not, we can use the selected herbal prescriptions above by Wu Jutang for the moist/greasy tongue condition.

It should be stressed that eventually the body *will* find its way, and the role of the practitioner is to recognize this tendency and assist appropriately. It is always wise to let the body struggle a little to find its way, especially in children. It is bad practice in 3E to intervene prematurely. What we read clinically as symptoms only represent the body's attempt to heal itself. (These principles are similar to the practice of homeopathy.)

It is important to note that causes of dampness and lingering of dampness may come not only from the external environment but from food, fluids, and/or stress. Today, especially in large, urban environments with hot and humid weather, air conditioners are used frequently. In the morning, before they are turned on, there is usually a damp smell in these environments. One way of dispersing this type of dampness is to use good quality incense prior to using air conditioning. Incense helps to rid the atmosphere of pathogens with the release of volatile oils that expel these factors.

It is also important to note that in damp heat environments we tend to crave and want to drink cold or ice cold drinks and eat damp foods, greasy foods, deep fried foods, spicy foods, dairy rich foods (e.g. ice cream), and caffeine. Bad practices such as eating late at night, and having sex on a full Stomach or whilst intoxicated, causes stagnation of food leading to lingering pathogens. All the above factors need to be eliminated, especially during the waiting period over the time intervals as outlined above.

Thin, yellow and dry tongue coating

After 24–72 hours, the body is now trying to perspire, *or* the patient presents with thin, yellow and dry tongue coating, and:

Pulse: slippery/rapid/large/full.

Symptoms: fever, aversion to heat, profuse sweating, thirst with a desire to drink cold beverages.

In this case we proceed to help the body with the *perspiration and heat purging* method.

Gui Zhi decoction with *Shi Gao* and *Zhi Mu* has a much stronger effect on providing nutritive essence than *Bai Hu Tang*, the formula of choice in Wen Bing Xue's *Warm Disease Theory*. However, we are following the same *principle* by combining the nourishing and heat-clearing effect through the addition of *Shi Gao* and *Zhi Mu* to give *Gui Zhi Tang Jia with Shi Gao and Zhi Mu*.

Gui Zhi	10 gm
Bai Shao	10 gm
Ginger	10 gm
Da Zao	7 pieces (to support Stomach and Spleen with *Shi Gao* and *Zhi Mu*)

Zhi Gan Cao	6 gm
Shi Gao	20–30 gm (prepared earlier)
Zhi Mu	5–8 gm

This treatment is prepared by boiling 5 cups of water and adding Shi Gao (pulverized) first. When there are approximately 3–3½ cups of water left from boiling add the rest of the prescription until one cup of the infusion remains for consumption.

For wheezing and heavy cough with or without perspiration add:

Ma Huang (ephedra) 9–12 gm

Xing Ren 7–9 gm.

Lingering fever

For lingering fever use the Wu Jutang Method of *clearing heat and draining fire* (Wen and Seifert 2000, p.83).

Bitter, cold medicinals directly clear internal heat, and clear and discharge pathogenic Fire for conditions of smoldering heat confined in the Qi aspect that transforms into Fire. This condition causes symptoms of lingering fever, vexation and agitation, bitter taste in the mouth, thirst, dark yellow urine, red tongue, and yellow tongue moss. Its paradigmatic formula is Coptis Toxin-Resolving Decoction (*Huang Lian Jie Du Tang*).

Note that this Qi-clearing method cannot be used until after warm disease external patterns have been resolved. Inappropriate application of such "cold" and "cooling" medicines may effectively cause "freezing," resulting in the concealment of disease pathogens rather than their resolution.

Thus, cold and cooling Qi-clearing medicinals are contraindicated when damp heat lingers in the Qi aspect.

Caution must also be used when applying the Qi-clearing method on patients with pre-existing Yang vacuity. This problem is addressed in the 3E Herbal Method by adding a large dose of *Shi Gao* to *Gui Zhi Tang* in order to support upright Yang.

Finally, fever and pathogens can also linger due to inappropriate diet and lifestyle and, as mentioned earlier, patients must abstain from these behaviours during the treatments.

Thick yellow coating on tongue

Da Chen Qi Tang is the principal formula (the same choice as Wu Jutang) to purge damp/heat and toxins using bitter, cold and down-bearing herbs, using the purgation method.

The 3E Method agrees with Wu Jutang, according to Wen and Seifert (2000, p.89).

1. *Clearing bowels and discharging heat* method uses bitter, cold, down-bearing medicinals to drain repletion heat from the intestinal bowels when heat transfers to Yang brightness and binds internally, causing symptoms such as tidal fever, delirious speech, constipation, hard abdominal distention that refuses pressure, old yellow tongue moss (or in severe cases scorched-black tongue moss with thorns), and sunken replete pulse. Its paradigmatic formulas are Greater Qi-Infusing Decoction (*Da Cheng Qi Tang*) and Stomach-Regulating Qi-Infusing Decoction (*Tiao WeiCheng Qi Tang*).

2. *Coursing stagnation and clearing stools* method clears accumulations and stagnations, and also discharges confined heat below. It is generally used for accumulations and stagnations of damp heat that combine and bind in the Stomach and intestines, causing symptoms such as dilations and fullness in the gastro-abdominal region, nausea and vomiting, turbid yellow-brown diarrhea, and yellow tongue moss. Its paradigmatic formula is Unripe

Bitter Orange Stagnation-Abducting Decoction (*Zhi Shi Dao Zhi Tang*).

When the Qi dynamic has bonded with the pathogen and the body is trying to purge via the intestines, this will be reflected by:

Pulse: large, deep, strong, or forceful.

Tongue: thick yellow coating.

Symptoms: tidal fever, delirious speech, constipation, hard abdominal distention that refuses pressure, old yellow tongue moss, or in severe cases scorched-black tongue moss with thorns (Wen and Seifert 2000, p.88).

3. *Clearing stasis and breaking binds* method breaks and scatters lower burner blood stasis accumulation and binding by downward-through clearing. It is generally prescribed when blood accumulation in the lower burner results from stasis and heat binding together during a warm disease, causing symptoms of distention, fullness and acute pain in the lower abdomen, constipation (but normal urination), manic behavior, rinsing of the mouth without desire to drink, crimson-purple tongue, and fine replete pulse. Its paradigmatic formula is Peach Kernel Qi-Infusing Decoction (*Tao Ren Cheng Qi Tang*).

This condition can be seen in patients undergoing chemotherapy and radiation therapy, and in trauma, longstanding diseases with retention and old age.

The *downward-through clearing* method, particularly the bitter, cold, downward-through clearing method, is one of the most effective treatments for warm diseases.

Li Bao Yi pointed out its importance when he explained: "The Stomach is the sea of the five viscera and the six bowels; it occupies the middle Earth, and it readily collects and stores." Pathogenic heat that enters the Stomach does not transfer, and when warm disease heat binds in the Stomach bowel, the *downward-through clearing* method yields results in 60 to 70 percent of all cases. Applying downward-through clearing prematurely is not a serious mistake in a warm disease.

In clinical practice, different combinations are used for different patient conditions. It is common for both the *downward-through clearing* and *reinforcing* methods to be used together. The simultaneous use of the *downward-through clearing* and *right-Qi-assisting* method is a widespread practice, suitable for Yang brightness bowel repletions with right Qi vacuity. In bowel repletion accompanied by Yin fluid vacuity, the *downward-through clearing* method is combined with the *Yin-nourishing* method. Downward-through clearing can also be combined with *Lung-diffusing, orifice-opening,* or *six-bowel clearing and coursing* to treat Yang brightness bowel repletions with phlegm heat obstructing the Lung, pathogens blocking the Pericardium, or binding of Small Intestine heat, respectively.

Note that the *downward-through clearing* method is contraindicated in cases of repletion where warm disease pathogens have already transferred to the interior but internal binding has not occurred (i.e. where pathogenic heat or damp heat is without form).

It must be used cautiously when right Qi is vacuous and weak. This method must be combined with the reinforcing method when pathogens are replete and the right Qi is vacuous. Purge only when the tongue coating is yellow.

Constipation that develops during the final stage of a warm disease occurs because the fluids are desiccated and the intestines are drying out. Therefore, the bitter, cold, downward-through clearing method is contraindicated (Wen and Seifert 2000, p.90).

Note the example above refers to conditions where there is Yin injury or Yin consumption due to heat in the intestines in the case of a warm disease. However, this condition may also arise from constitutional Yin deficiency where heat has consumed all the fluid and Yin in the intestines. The formula used in this case should nourish Yin/fluid as the main focus and also clear any heat and encourage bowel movement.

The tongue will be dry/red with or without cracks, as the Yin and fluids have been consumed. The body has weakened, and the pulse will be forceless/fine. In this case use *Zeng Yi Tang*, or *Zeng Yi Cheng Qi Tang*.

Zeng Yi Tang is used for acute cases, and if there is no response within 12 hours, use *Zeng Yi Cheng Qi Tang* (Bensky and Barolet 1990).

Ying construction level

The pathogen in this case has passed through and/or overpowered the Wei and Qi levels, and started to attack the Ying construction level of the body. The nutritive fluid aspect of the life-force energy of the body is being attacked and consumed. The tongue becomes red, and the pulse becomes fine and rapid.

Pulse: usually fine, rapid.

Tongue: body is deep crimson red, thorny, cracked, there is little
coating.

There are usually 3 characteristics of *pulse* in Ying-construction level sickness due to warmth:

- If rapid/thready/fine, the pathogen is lodged in the Ying level generally.

- If wiry/rapid and full/rapid, the pathogen is lodged in the Pericardium.

- If wiry/rapid and weak/empty, the pathogen is lodged in the Liver.

GENERAL YING CONSTRUCTION METHODS

1. *Clearing-construction and discharging-heat* method induces transference and resolution of pathogenic Qi from the construction to the Qi aspect, using medicinals to clear and resolve construction aspect heat pathogens in combination with light-clearing, thrusting-out, discharging medicinals. It is prescribed when heat enters the construction aspect,

causing symptoms such as fever that intensifies at night, vexation, insomnia, delirious speech, rashes that have only partially surfaced, and crimson tongue. Its paradigmatic formula is Construction-Clearing Decoction (*Qing Ying Tang*) (Wen and Seifert 2000, p.91).

2. *Clearing both Qi and construction* method couples construction-clearing with Qi-clearing medicinals, and is used for pathogens entering the construction with Qi heat remaining exuberant (i.e. for patterns of intensifying of heat at both the Qi and construction), causing symptoms of vigorous fever, strong thirst, vexation, macula spots that have surfaced to the exterior, crimson tongue, and dry yellow tongue moss. Generally, formulas like Jade Lady Variant Brew (*Jia Jian Yu Nu Jian*) are prescribed.

    The *construction-clearing* method is usually coupled with the *Qi-clearing* method in practice, sometimes also being combined with other methods, such as the *orifice-opening* method or *wind-extinguishing* method.

Note that this method is contraindicated if the pathogen has lodged in the Qi aspect, without having entered the construction aspect, although internal heat may be very strong—if used erroneously it may guide deep entry of pathogenic Qi.

Pathogens cannot successfully be transferred to the Qi aspect when they have first entered the construction but not yet stirred the blood. They cannot be resolved using only medicinals that clear and cool the construction-blood—those that thrust out and discharge must also be used. Isolated use of construction-clearing, heat-discharging medicinals will not be successful even when pathogens have entered the blood, and they must be concurrently supplemented with those that cool and that dissipate the blood (Wen and Seifert 2000, p.91).

Therefore, if the tongue coat is yellow/dry with red body use *Jia Jian Yu Nu Jian*. In the 3E Herbal Method we would use *Gui Zhi Tang* with *Shi Gao* (30–60 gm) and *Zhi Mu* (5–10 gm). If there is no coat, and the tongue is red or crimson or worse, use *Qing Ying Tang*.

PERICARDIUM AND HEART: YING LEVEL METHODS

The orifice-opening method

This treatment method clears the mind by opening and clearing through the Heart orifices to transform phlegm, thrust out the network vessels with aromatic medicinals, open closures, and through-clear the orifices. It is used when warm disease pathogens close the Pericardium and cloud the spirit or cause coma. In clinical practice, there are two major subdivisions of this method.

1. *Clearing the Heart and opening the orifices* method clarifies the mind by clearing and discharging pathogenic heat from the Pericardium, and transforming phlegm and out-thrusting the network vessels when warm disease heat counterflows into the Pericardium and blocks the Heart orifices, creating symptoms such as cold limbs, clouded spirit (the mind being sometimes clear and sometimes confused) with delirious speech (or coma without speech), sluggish tongue, and vivid-crimson tongue. Commonly-used formulas include Peaceful Palace Bovine Bezoar Pill (*An Gong Niu Huang Wan*), Supreme Jewel Elixir (*Zhi Bao Dan*), and Purple Snow Elixir (*Zi Xue Dan*).

2. *Sweeping phlegm and opening the orifices* method diffuses the orifices and opens closures by clearing and transforming both damp heat and turbid phlegm, and is suitable for use when confined, steaming damp heat ferments into turbid phlegm, which clouds the mind and closes the clear orifices, causing symptoms such as clouded spirit with delirious speech, red tongue, and sticky slimy yellow moss. Its paradigmatic formula is Acorus and Curuma Decoction (*Chang Pu Yu Jin Tang*).

The *orifice-opening* method is used by itself during *emergencies* to alleviate clouded spirit, but is otherwise almost always used with supplementary methods. The *Heart-clearing orifice-opening* method, for example, is normally used together with the *construction-clearing, blood cooling, wind-extinguishing,* or *desertion-stemming* methods, while the *phlegm-sweeping, orifice-opening* method is normally used with the *heat-clearing* or *dampness-transforming* methods.

The orifice-opening method is contraindicated when clouded spirit is attributable to exuberant Qi aspect heat.

The Heart-clearing, orifice-opening method cannot be used even when pathogens enter the construction-blood, unless they cause closure and reversal.

The functions of the Heart-clearing, orifice-opening and phlegm-sweeping, orifice-opening methods are different, and clinically they are used for different patterns and must not be confused. For treatment of warm diseases, since the orifice-opening method is used only as an emergency treatment, appropriate supplementary methods must be applied according to the relative strength and weakness of the right and pathogenic Qi, as reflected in the clinical expressions (Wen and Seifert 2000, pp.93–94).

LIVER YING LEVEL METHODS

The wind-extinguishing method

The *wind-extinguishing* method for internal stirring of Liver wind in warm disease extinguishes Liver wind and controls tetanic reversal to settle fright and stop tetanic spasms. Its use with convulsions or tetanic reversals in clinical practice is subdivided into two primary methods.

1. *Cooling the Liver and extinguishing wind* method acts principally to clear heat and cool the Liver, extinguish wind, and stop tetanic spasms. It is applicable when there is intensification of warm disease-causing heat pathogens, stirring Liver wind internally, causing symptoms of scorching body heat, cold limbs, intermittent tetanic spasms of the limbs (in severe

cases), arched-back rigidity, clouded spirit without speech, and string-like rapid pulse. Its paradigmatic formula is Antelope Horn and Uncaria Decoction (*Ling Jiao Gou Teng Tang*).

2. *Nourishing Yin and extinguishing wind* method extinguishes vacuity wind by fostering Yin and subduing Yang. The method is suitable for the late stages of warm disease when the true Yin is depleted and damaged, the Liver loses nourishment, and vacuity wind stirs internally, causing symptoms such as trembling of the hands and feet, convulsions (in severe cases), cold limbs, lassitude of the spirit, crimson tongue, scant tongue moss, and vacuous fine pulse. Its paradigmatic formula is Major Wind-Stabilizing Pill (*Da Ding Feng Zhu*).

The *wind-extinguishing* method is suitable for treating tetanic reversals, but is seldom used alone. The *liver-cooling, wind-extinguishing* method is normally combined with the *Qi-clearing, construction-clearing, blood-cooling*, or *downward-through clearing* methods, depending on the nature of the pathogen. The *Yin-nourishing, wind-extinguishing* method is normally combined with the *Qi-boosting, desertion-stemming, blood-quickening*, or *phlegm-transforming* methods.

The *Liver-cooling, wind-extinguishing* and the *Yin-nourishing, wind-extinguishing* methods are very different. In the former, the focus is on eliminating the pathogens; in the latter, on assisting the right Qi. Clinically, therefore, distinctions must be made as to whether moving wind is replete or vacuous.

In children suffering from warm diseases with pathogens in the defense and Qi aspects, convulsions may develop very quickly due to the accompanying high fever. The principal treatment remains to clear the heat and thrust out the pathogens. Convulsions recede as soon as fevers reduce. Thus, *Liver-cooling, wind-extinguishing* medicinals must not be used too early (Wen and Seifert 2000, pp.94–95).

139

XUE BLOOD LEVEL METHODS

In these cases the pathogen has penetrated the depths of the body and disperses into the blood and severe damage occurs. The tongue becomes *dark* red, the pulse becomes thin and racing, fluids and Yin are consumed rapidly, and Yang is threatened.

The blood-cooling method

This method uses clearing and cooling medicinals to clear and disperse blood aspect heat toxin pathogens to cool blood and nourish Yin, clear Fire and resolve toxins, through-clear the network vessels, and scatter blood, principally when warm disease pathogenic heat enters deeply into the blood aspect, causing strong heat toxins, damaged network vessels, and stirring blood patterns. Clinically, there are two major subdivisions.

1. *Cooling and scattering blood* method cools and resolves blood aspect heat pathogens, quickens, and scatters blood. It is suitable when heat enters the blood aspect and exuberant heat stirs the blood, causing symptoms such as scorching heat, agitation or mania (in severe cases), delirious speech, vomiting of blood, nose bleeding, blood in the stools, blood in the urine, concentrated rashes, and dark crimson tongue. Its paradigmatic formula is Rhinoceros Horn and Rehmannia Decoction (*Xi Jiao Di Huang Tang*).

2. *Clearing Qi and blood with large doses* method uses large doses of heat-clearing, toxin-resolving medicinals to clear and disperse Qi and blood aspect "triple burner" heat toxins for congested exuberant warm disease heat toxins that force Qi and blood to overflow and spread through the "triple burner," causing symptoms such as vigorous fever, stabbing headache, thirst, foul mouth odor, visual distortion, delirious speech, mania, bone and joint aches, backache (in which the back feels like it has been dealt a crushing blow), purple-black rashes, or nosebleeds, or

blood in the urine, dry yellow or scorched-black tongue moss, and purple tongue. Its paradigmatic prescription is Scourge-Clearing Toxin-Vanquishing Beverage (*Qing Wen Bai Du Yin*).

The *blood-cooling* method is normally combined with the *orifice-opening* method, the *wind-extinguishing* method, or the *blood-quickening, stasis-transforming* methods.

Note that it is premature to use the *blood-cooling* method even after heat has entered the construction aspect, unless it is stirring the blood. However, *blood-quickening, stasis-scattering* medicinals must be used without delay when non-stop bleeding occurs after intensifying blood heat causes stasis and stagnation in the network vessels.

Clinical considerations should not be limited to *defense Qi-construction-blood* theory when warm disease heat toxins force overflowing, internally and externally, above and below. In such cases, large doses of *clearing and resolving* medicinals must be used to strongly clear the Qi and blood, drain the Fire, and resolve the toxins (Wen and Seifert 2000, pp.92–93).

This presentation completes the four levels of Wen Bing.

The remainder of this chapter is based upon *Warm Disease Theory* (Wen and Seifert 2000, pp.96–99).

The Yin-nourishing method

This method nourishes and supplements Yin humor, and is generally used when warm disease heat pathogens are gradually resolving and Yin humor is damaged, as its main functions are to nourish and supplement true Yin, to engender liquid and nourish humor, and to moisten dryness and control Fire. Warm disease heat pathogens can easily detriment and damage fluids. They are particularly liable to damage liquid and consume humor during the final stages of a disease. The degree of damage to the Yin humor is closely related to the patient's prognosis.

The physicians of ancient times postulated, "For one part fluid there is one part engendering-dynamic." As this statement suggests, the Yin-nourishing method is commonly used in the treatment of warm diseases. Clinically, the Yin-nourishing method is divided into three primary approaches, according to its different body functions.

1. *Nourishing the Lungs and Stomach* method uses sweet cold moisturizing medicinals to nourish Lung and Stomach fluids. It is suitable when heat damages the Yin humor of the Stomach and then begins to gradually resolve, causing symptoms such as dryness of mouth, nose, lip, and throat, dry coughing with scant phlegm, and dry tongue moss. Its paradigmatic formula is Adenophora/Glehnia and Ophiopogon Decoction (*Sha Shen Mai Men Dong Tang*).

2. *Increasing humor and moisturizing the intestines* method uses sweet and salty cold medicinals to engender liquid and nourish humor, moisten the intestines, and through-clear stools. It is generally used when heat pathogens have damaged Yin humor, desiccated liquid, and dried the intestines, leaving symptoms such as constipation, dry mouth and throat, and dry red tongue. Its paradigmatic formula is Humor-Increasing Decoction (*Zeng Ye Tang*).

3. *Nourishing and supplementing Kidney Yin* method uses sweet cold nourishing-moisturizing medicinals to supplement true Yin, strengthen Water, and subdue Yang. It is generally prescribed when lingering warm heat pathogens rob and scorch the true Yin, creating increased vacuity diminished pathogen patterns, causing symptoms including fever, red complexion, more heat in the palms and soles than in the back of the hands and top of the feet, dry mouth and throat, lassitude of the spirit, desire to sleep, palpitations (sometimes), crimson tongue with scant moss, and a vacuous, fine or bounding, regularly interrupted pulse.

Its paradigmatic formula is Pulse Restorative Variant Decoction (*Jia Jian Fu Mai Tang*).

Pulse Restorative Variant Decoction (*Jia Jian Fu Mai Tang*) nourishes the Yin and reinforces the blood, clears heat, and restores the pulse. It is used to treat conditions that occur following warm heat diseases, in which residual pathogenic heat lingers and Yin-fluids are damaged (hence increased vacuity diminished pathogen patterns).

The *Yin-nourishing* method has a wide range of applications in the treatment of warm diseases, and can be used with a large number of other treatment methods. It can be appropriate variously to nourish Yin and resolve the exterior, to nourish Yin and clear heat, to nourish Yin and downward-through clear, or to nourish Yin and extinguish wind.

However, Yin-nourishing is contraindicated whenever warm disease pathogenic heat is exuberant because if used erroneously it causes the pathogen to lodge, and must be used with due caution whenever damp heat patterns are being treated, or else pathogens may become adhesive and very difficult to resolve.

The desertion-securing method

This method is an emergency rectification measure used for vacuity desertion. This method encompasses the *Yang-returning, counterflow-stemming*, and the *Qi-boosting, desertion-securing* methods, which are generally prescribed clinically for the critical conditions of Yang collapse, reversal, counterflow, and sudden desertion of right Qi. These unusual changes of Yang collapse and Qi desertion do not normally follow, although Yin vacuity occurs quite commonly in warm diseases. These changes generally eventuate only if the Yin has been suddenly damaged during the development of a disease—a predicament that can be caused by either vacuity of right Qi with overabundance of pathogenic Qi, or abuse of sweat-inducing and downward-through clearing methods. The clinical situation becomes critical in such cases, so the *Yang-returning, counterflow-stemming* or *Qi-boosting, desertion-stemming* methods must be used, as discussed below.

1. *Boosting Qi and securing desertion* method boosts Qi and engenders fluids, stops sweating and secures desertion. It is normally used when, during the course of a warm disease, the Qi and Yin have both been damaged and the right Qi is verging on desertion and there are symptoms such as profuse sweating, shortness of breath, lassitude, exhaustion, and fine pulse without strength. Its paradigmatic formula is Pulse-Engendering Powder (*Sheng Mai San*).

2. *Returning Yang and stemming counterflow* method uses acrid, hot medicinals to rouse Yang in cases of sudden desertion of Yang Qi with symptoms of cold extremities, dribbling sweat, expiration of spirit, curled up posture (fetal position), white complexion, and fine faint pulse that has nearly expired. Its paradigmatic formula is Ginseng, Aconite, Dragon Bone, and Oyster Shell Decoction (*Shen Fu Long Mu Tang*).

In clinical practice these two methods are normally used together. They are further generally coupled with *orifice-opening* methods in conditions of internal closure with external desertion.

The *desertion-stemming* method is normally used only in critical conditions; therefore, when used, it must be used without delay. Also, the number of doses per day, the time between doses, and the strength of doses must be understood. Likewise, the patient's rapidly-changing condition needs to be closely monitiored so that beneficial modifications can be made. The importance of monitoring the patient in Wan's 3E Method can not be emphasized enough.

As an emergency treatment, the *desertion-stemming* method must be used only when appropriate and then discontinued immediately. As soon as desertion stops and the Yang returns clinical pattern identification and treatment determination must be performed quickly according to the patient's rapidly-evolving condition.

LINGERING DAMPNESS AFTER YANG DESERTION

When we are able to rescue a patient from desertion patterns (as above), it is highly likely that damp pathogens will linger in the weakened body. These damp pathogens are capable of literally "sticking" around. As per the Yin and Yang, a hot disease can turn into a cold pattern and vice versa. At this point, the focus of treatment is to rebuild the patient's immunity and strength, and some changes will need to be implemented to ensure success.

Strengthening a weakened body recovering from a warm disease is not an easy task particularly when the Yin and Yang of the body has become exhausted. It is wise to start with a formula that will strengthen Qi (acquired vital energy) and to clear the body of lingering pathogens. Picture an old steam train, where the coal needs to keep getting shoveled into the burner for the train to keep moving. In this sense acquired vital energy has a similar function—to keep the body moving.

The recovering patient should abstain from:

- alcohol
- cigarette smoking
- cold or raw food
- dairy products
- ice cold drinks
- overconsumption of fluids
- starch rich diet
- sweets—ice cream, candy, rich desserts
- too many diuretics
- too much caffeine.

DAMP FROM DEFICIENCY AND/OR LINGERING PATHOGENS

Main symptoms: body feels heavy, stifling sensation in the chest, epigastric pain.

Pulse: soggy, soft, weak.

Tongue: slimy, moist coating (whether white or yellow), pale and/or flabby.

3E formula of choice

A good formula to consider as a base formula for any kind of damp and strengthening the middle or acquired Qi is *Er Chen Tang*.

Ban Xia	10 gm
Chen Pi	12 gm
Fu Ling	10 gm
Zhi Can Gao	6 gm

When the patient feels better, the appetite is returning, pulse is strengthening, daily activities are slowly resuming, and stools return to normal, then we can assume the damp pathogens have been sufficiently cleared to use a formula such as *Ba Zhen Tang* (others of a similar nature can also be used) as the focus is then to nourish, replenish, and restore the body to good health.

CONCLUSION: TO THE PHYSICIAN

A few final words...

Healing is not just a lifestyle—it's a way of life; it is not just being technically proficient: good at needling or determining and deciding what the dosage of a herb should be. To heal in the correct manner one ought to live in a healing manner also. Below are some suggestions of rules to live by, in order to help develop the healing method to deeper levels. Wan believes 3E physicians are obliged to follow this path.

Self-work

A practitioner should always practice what she or he preaches. Hypocrisy has a short life in authentic practice. Self-awareness and the continuing development of one's own concentration and skillful thinking practices are essential to becoming a "superior" physician.

Meditation is important to calm the mind, and to deepen one's concentration during treatment. A good website to visit is www. vbgnet.org (accessed February 2011). I cannot stress enough the need for constant meditation and awareness practice. A Wan's 3E physician strives for mental tranquility, harmony, and inner happiness above all. A good place to start is with breath counting meditation; then learn about the various methods, in particular the "Anapanasati" method taught by the Buddha.

Practice breath counting at least 2–3 times a week for a minimum of 15 minutes to begin with and go from there. Usually breath counting is a good place to start. For more information on this please visit www.accesstoinsight.org (accessed February 2011).

Meditation is one part of the many factors for self-work. Contemplation on the teaching, practicing virtues such as generosity, respect for one's teacher and taking care regarding not to indulge in: alcohol and drugs, sleep, overworking, anger, hatred, delusion, sex.

All the above tax ability and capability to gain insight and deep awareness. Wan's 3E physicians need to be sharp, alert, and mindful at all times in speech, thought, and action.

Social charity: Giving

Practice generosity, by donating time, money, and/or food, and better still all of the above, to charity and/or the community on a regular basis. In terms of donating money to charity, at least 10 percent of one's weekly income is sufficient. It is good to spread healing and happiness to others, especially to those in need and also to support the Sangha community of monks. You can find out where your local Sangha community of monks is by simply searching on Google for a Theravadin monastery in your area or state.

Giving to the community is a good practice; volunteering at homeless shelters, foodbanks, and when there is a natural disaster or a man-made crisis is essential to develop a giving, compassionate nature. A Wan's 3E physician strives to abide in the Divine Abidings as mentioned by the Buddha: loving kindness to all beings, compassion to all beings, gladness in other people's success, and equanimity to all beings.

Discover, in other words, the practice of Metta, which translates as "loving kindness," the cultivation of which is a popular form of meditation in Buddhism. Find out more about this practice and strive for it daily.

Giving back to the profession

The Chinese medicine and acupuncture profession needs your help! If the profession grows, the practitioners will grow. Extending oneself into the practice acupuncture community gives support to other practitioners and also creates a community from which the public can benefit. Join your local acupuncture society or organization, attend their functions, stay informed about what is happening in the community.

Knowledge sharing: Teaching

It is good to share one's experiences and knowledge with other practitioners, particularly if it also helps to improve treatment ability and effectiveness.

Wan's 3E physicians are required to teach at some point at least for a period of time. Wan's 3E physicians are permitted to teach only after practicing the Method for five years.

Respect for one's teacher

In the tradition of most good schools it is always proper to show respect to one's teacher. A good teacher is hard to find in any aspect of life, and if one is lucky enough to do so, one must always show respect for the teacher.

Many students these days expect to be taught without giving anything in return or without going through any testing, but in the lineage of true Taoist teachers, students are chosen according to their motivation, intent, and ability to let go of ego as a first prerequisite. A good teacher knows when a student is suited to their teaching style, but in the university method, it doesn't matter. Once a student pays the tuition fee the institution is forced to "teach." The advantage of this, however, is that anyone can learn, and it removes the possibility of discrimination.

In terms of the Ancient method a teacher usually tests the student at the beginning, in the middle, and the end. Of course there are teachers that abuse this authority, but if the teacher is a good, true teacher, devoted to the welfare of others, it would be hard for that teacher to abuse their authority. However, it is true that some students are not suited to certain teachers' ways of teaching.

The age old method of apprenticeship has lost its popularity in the current community; however, in such a relationship, the student is endowed with the teacher's practical and clinical knowledge over a period of time. If well done, it is more valuable than any university degree, precious gems or metals. If the teaching is authentic and the student is accepting, many good things will come of it.

It is important for a student to always show respect to the teacher at the beginning, in the middle, and the end. Respect does not mean the practice of blind faith, though, nor just believing anything because the teacher said so. A good teacher welcomes questions and is eager to offer explanation. The practice of respect is a practice of humility and to show gratitude for the kindness and willingness of the teacher to teach, but this is seldom recognized these days. There are many good practitioners who do not teach. It is the same in any field. If one is lucky to receive good teaching, then one should show respect in all ways to the teacher for they are indeed fortunate.

To know if the teacher is good or if the teaching works is not something one can find out immediately, and is a difficult problem to overcome. Once the teachings have been applied over a period one will know whether the teaching is good. In Chinese medicine one can follow a teacher for many years, and sometimes be disappointed. This explains the importance and luck of receiving good teaching. If one is lucky and receives the correct teaching it saves the student much time and money and avoids searching endlessly.

Is paying a teacher bad?

Let me answer the question with a question: Should a student learn for free and offer no token in return? And does not the teacher need things in life like anyone else?

In Buddhism lay people offer food, clothing, and shelter to the monks, and in return the monks offer insight and the invaluable, timeless, and most precious of all Dhamma teachings of the Buddha.

Exchange is a two-way street.

In ancient societies, whether it be Vedic, Brahmin, Hindu, Buddhism, Taoism, etc., respect, giving or offering or tokens to one's teacher was seen as a virtuous practice, and in return, the teacher gave precious teachings.

I wish you much Metta, and urge that you strive for skillful thinking and behavior. May it be profitable in all ways to yourself and everyone around you.

Giorgio Repeti

APPENDIX: BUDDHISM, TAOISM, AND GENERAL THOUGHTS ON CURING AND HEALING

Buddha's Eightfold Path

Ethical conduct (sila):

- Right Speech.

- Right Action.

- Right Livelihood.

Mental development:

- Right Effort.

- Right Mindfulness.

- Right Concentration.

Wisdom:

- Right View.

- Right Intention.

Right View is not limited to medicine or healing but rather to the human condition of "dukkha": suffering and samsara, which translates as "continuous flowing," and refers to the cycle of birth, life, death, and rebirth in Buddhism, as the reality of life as it is.

We use this application of Right View of the human condition in the clinic to establish the Right Intention, thus facilitating "Right Action" in treatment.

Although it is desirable to achieve the entire Eightfold Path we will not discuss the complete discipline in this book.

Buddha broke down the body into 32 elements:

1. *Kesaa ca*—Hair of the head

2. *Lomaa ca*—Hair of the body

3. *Nakhaa ca*—Nails

4. *Dantaa ca*—Teeth

5. *Taco ca*—Skin

6. *Ma.msañca*—Flesh

7. *Nhaaruu ca*—Tendons

8. *A.t.thii ca*—Bones

9. *A.t.thimiñjañca*—Bone marrow

10. *Vakkañca*—Spleen

11. *Hadayañca*—Heart

12. *Yakanañca*—Liver

13. *Kilomakañca*—Membranes

14. *Pihakañca*—Kidneys

15. *Papphaasañca*—Lungs

16. *Antañca*—Large Intestines

17. *Antagu.nañca*—Small Intestines

18. *Udariyañca*—Gorge

19. *Kariisañca*—Feces

20. *Matthalu"ngañca*—Brain

21. *Pittañca*—Gall

22. *Semhañca*—Phlegm

23. *Pubbo ca*—Lymph

24. *Lohitañca*—Blood

25. *Sedo ca*—Sweat

26. *Medo ca*—Fat

27. *Assu ca*—Tears

28. *Vasaa ca*—Oil

29. *Khe.lo ca*—Saliva

30. *Si"nghaa.nikaa ca*—Mucus

31. *Lasikaa ca*—Oil in the joints

32. *Muttañca*—Urine

(Dhammadharo 2010)

Buddha identified Four Detriments to health as:

- birth
- sickness
- old age
- death.

These Four Detriments are an inevitable part of life for everyone.

1. *Longevity and Vitality*: Dr. Wan quoted the Buddha extensively, and in reference to the four detriments stated clearly that sickness and old age can be significantly reduced with his healing method, even eliminated. This goal was an ambition and ideal for which he strove in his therapy.

2. *Balance and Flow*: Dr. Wan stated that the body has a natural flow and sequence, and thus treatment needs to help the body stay in that natural flow and sequence, through natural means.

3. *Perfection and Intervention*: Dr. Wan stated that in Taoism, as related to Chinese medicine and healing, there is the view that the body is perfect and needs little intervention.

4. *Divinity and Disease*: Dr. Wan quoted from "Huang Di Nei Jing Su Wen"—and in the *Golden Needle Wang Le Ting*: "When the righteous Qi arrives, there is no disease."

Does this last principle of divinity have relevance in the final stages of life when the natural state of dying, of passing, follows that of being alive? If the body is meant to decay, disrupt, breakdown, fall apart—what then is the role of the healer in this process? Can someone die without suffering in the final years? My answer is no.

Dis-ease as the word implies, is part of existence whether we like it or not. The practice of Chinese medicine is one that seeks to disable the "dis" and create more of the "ease."

The "reality" of the human body *is* decline and breakdown—nothing can prevent this.

Right View

Right View is right understanding of the human condition of dukkha. A good practitioner is aware of the "reality" of decline.

Many practitioners are tempted to form personal attachments to the results of treatment. It is important to remain detached and relaxed. Results are arbitrary and subjective in the "reality of decline."

The perception of prevention and cure surface in the reality as being only momentary, this perception is known as true awareness and insight.

We can treat conditions such as IBS or sore throat, temporarily, or for a long time (subjective). Then something else happens and so on and so on, but what remains true is that we will never be able to cure the human condition of dukkha with any medical treatment. The aim then is to constantly harmonize the *dis*.

I have noted a common thread between teachers who lay claim to be able to heal anything and everything. There is always an answer, there is always the right herb or acupuncture point, etc. This is true to an extent, however, even Buddha and Lao Tzu could not cheat death! Nor the aging process.

A practitioner needs to root his reality in this fact, to detach from the false reality of "savior," and to see themselves accurately as only a helper, one who helps to rid the *dis*.

Right Intention

Right Intention sees the limitations and barriers as well as all the possibilities that lie within those limitations and barriers. These parameters then set up the *Right Action*.

Right View has given us to understand the limitation that life has to end, that decay and breakdown is essential and is natural. Therefore what is the Intention of the practitioner in regards to the patient?

1. FOCUS

To harmonize the body at that given moment when a patient is lying on the treatment table (or wherever else). We go to work, analyzing, observing, inspecting, reflecting, feeling, listening, palpating, smelling, hearing. Then we observe the outcome through "solution consciousness" or the plan of treatment.

The plan of treatment is important. If the Right View with Right Intention and Right Action are not in their correct places, treatment will not be effective in that moment and can actually become a detriment to the patient. The sickness can become stronger and/or the body can be weakened as a result.

2. ROLE

If every person is destined to become old and frail and die what is the role of cure? What is the role of prevention? What are we curing, and what are we preventing? This is a central question for all health practitioners.

Our role is to assist the patient in leading a better, more harmonious life, and to guide him or her to avoid the pitfalls of a bad lifestyle and ill-health. But can we literary "save" their lives? What does this statement mean?

It is important to know one's domain or sphere of limitations. For example, acupuncture can do very little in a medical emergency such as the dismemberment of a limb. And acupressure can help with many issues that lie on the surface, but cannot cure skin cancer.

3. DIAGNOSIS

Correct diagnosis is crucial and without it, one's treatment will hardly be effective. The right diagnosis is not subjective, it is tangible and can be observed and measured.

With the correct diagnosis, the result will be correct treatment and the patient will feel better for a long period of time (or shorter, depending on the condition at hand). Moreover we *feel* the pulse, *see* the tongue, *observe* the complexion and *hear* from the patient, whether symptoms are changing for the better. The scientific tangibility of results is visible, heard and felt by the practitioner and experienced by the patient.

Often practitioners rely solely on patient feedback. In the 3E Method we have our instruments of testing and it is crucial for the practitioner to know factually and tangibly the results of the treatment.

4. AWARENESS (OR MINDFULNESS)

Right Intention is about one's awareness (mindfulness) at the moment of:

- diagnosis

- treatment

- professional life.

Taoist thought

Taoism formulates numerological sequences (can numerological sequences literally be "countless"?) to determine patterns and thus create a path of deeper understanding in the nature of disease. For example, an eight-year cycle for men, seven-year cycle for women, where there is a rise and decline.

Taoism has developed many numerological patterns in reference to birth, seasons, and treatments. A significant feature is that none of the sequences can be 100 percent accurate. One need only use the sequences as a general guide and then rely upon one's intuition, awareness, and wisdom.

Right View is that the destiny of all people is old age (unless life is cut short, of course).

General thoughts on curing and healing

Dr. Wan insisted that his method can resolve all sickness, but then how is it that some of his patients saw him regularly for over thirty years?

As I observed Dr. Wan in practice, as well as many other well-trained practitioners, I also asked the patients questions such as, "How long have you been seeing the practitioner." I also remember Dr. Wan mentioning that he had been seeing some patients for 30 years in Hong Kong.

I have now seen some patients for longer than five years. I correct some issues, then another arises, and so forth.

So what then is a "cure" from this perspective? Is there such a thing? In my observations thus far, I don't believe that cure is the correct word. We help patients live a more comfortable life, but there is no "cure" for life, from birth, for even Buddha said that death is caused by "birth."

However, if healing for the human condition of suffering exists, it is called *nibbana*. At the time of writing this text, it remains something that one day I hope we can achieve.

Buddha himself could not stop the body becoming old and ill! How many masters or doctors can prevent themselves getting old or falling prey to sickness? How many health practitioners themselves would authentically provide a role model for health, emotional maturity, or spiritual mastery?

Improving the patient's chances of having less illness in the future marginally depends upon what you, as an aware and mindful practitioner, do in the present moment...

We can help "guide" our patients to a better tomorrow; however, the myriad of factors that affect health cannot be controlled in the clinic or by the practitioner. Emotions, attachments, greed, hatred, hunger, desire for worldliness, dissatisfaction, love issues, over-eating, indulgence and so on, and so on are factors that are beyond the control of practitioners' healing hands. The patient is thus responsible for most factors, and it is the responsibility of the practitioner, under the "duty of care," to be realistic about boundaries and limitations.

Having said all this—the 3E Method in turn can achieve much healing, but a practitioner needs to be aware of the delusions of "cure alls," "miracle herbs," and other inauthentic claims.

BIBLIOGRAPHY

Bensky, D. and Barolet, R. (1990) *Chinese Herbal Medicine Formulas and Strategies*. Vista, CA: Eastland Press.

Cheng Tsai Liu, Lui Zheng Cai and Ka Hua (1999) *A Study of Daoist Acupuncture and Moxibustion*. Boulder, CO: Blue Poppy Press.

Dhammadharo, A.L. (2010) *The Divine Mantra*, transl. Thanissaro Bhikhu. Available at www.accesstoinsight.org/lib/thai/lee/divinemantra.html, accessed 10 September 2010.

Huang Di Nei Jing Su Wen (1979) "Plain Questions." The Yellow Emperor's Classic of Internal Medicine. Beijing: People's Health Publishing House.

Huang Di Nei Jing Ling Shu (1979) "Miraculous Pivot." The Yellow Emperor's Classic of Internal Medicine. Beijing: People's Health Publishing House.

Huang Fu Mi (2007) *The Systematic Classic of Acupuncture and Moxibustion*. Boulder, CO: Blue Poppy Press.

Hui Chan Yu and Fu Ru Han (1997) *Golden Needle Wang Le-ting: A 20th Century Master's Approach to Acupuncture*. Boulder, CO: Blue Poppy Press.

Maciocia, G. (2000) "Articles—The Treatment of Respiratory Infections." Available at www.Giovanni-maciocia.com/articles/flu.html, accessed 11 January 2011.

Smith, J.M. (2007) *Genetic Roulette: The Documented Health Risks of Genetically Engineered Food*. White River Junction, Vermont: Chelsea Green Publishing.

Wen, J.M. and Seifert, G. (2000) *Warm Disease Theory: Wen Bing Xue*. Brookline, MA: Paradigm Publications.

Yifan Yang (2002) *Chinese Herbal Medicines: Comparisons and Characteristics*. Oxford: Churchill Livingstone.